NURSE **REPORT SHEET**

NURES/RECORDER INFO	
NAME	
ADDRESS	
PHONE	
NOTES	

EMERGENCY CONTACT	
NAME	
ADDRESS	
PHONE	
NOTES	

NAME	
ADDRESS	
PHONE	
NOTES	

We Would Appreciate Your BRIEF Review
on AMAZON.
Thank You.

Room:	Name:		Age/Sex:	Admit:
Code:	Allergies:			Isolation:

Attending:	Consults:

Diagnosis:	PMH:

Na:	RBC:	Meds:
K:	WBC:	
Ca:	Hgb:	
Mg:	Hct:	
Ph:	Platelets:	
Cl:	INR:	
Glu:	PTT:	
CO_2:	BUN:	
	Creat:	

Diagnostics:	IV:	Fluids:

Vitals:			Intake	Output
T:				
P:				
R:				
BP:				
O2:				

Neuro:	Neuro/CIWA	Cardio/Tele:	Pain Assess:	Pain Reassess:	Blood Sugar:
Resp:	Lungs/O2	DVT Prophylaxis:			
GI: Diet: Last BM:		Skin:	Edema:	Notes:	
GU:			Mobility:		

| Assessment | Education | IV's/Lines | Care plan review | I&O's | Chart check |
| Reassessment | Treatments | Skin | Nursing goals | General care | Sign off |

Room:	Name:		Age/Sex:	Admit:

Code:	Allergies:	Isolation:

Attending:	Consults:

Diagnosis:	PMH:

Na: **RBC:**   **Meds:**

K: **WBC:**

Ca: **Hgb:**

Mg: **Hct:**

Ph: **Platelets:**

Cl: **INR:**

Glu: **PTT:**

CO2:   **BUN:**

Creat:

Diagnostics:	IV:	Fluids:

Vitals:			Intake	Output

T:

P:

R:

BP:

O2:

Neuro: Neuro/CIWA	Cardio/Tele:	Pain Assess:	Pain Reassess:	Blood Sugar:

Resp: Lungs/O2

DVT Prophylaxis:

GI:
   Diet:
   Last BM:

GU:

Skin:	Edema:	Notes:
	Mobility:	

Assessment	Education	IV's/Lines	Care plan review	I&O's	Chart check
Reassessment	Treatments	Skin	Nursing goals	General care	Sign off

Room:	Name:		Age/Sex:	Admit:
Code:	Allergies:			Isolation:

Attending:	Consults:

Diagnosis:	PMH:

Na:	RBC:	Meds:
K:	WBC:	
Ca:	Hgb:	
Mg:	Hct:	
Ph:	Platelets:	
Cl:	INR:	
Glu:	PTT:	
CO2:	BUN:	
	Creat:	

Diagnostics:	IV:	Fluids:

Vitals:			Intake	Output
T:				
P:				
R:				
BP:				
O2:				

Neuro:	Neuro/CIWA	Cardio/Tele:	Pain Assess:	Pain Reassess:	Blood Sugar:
Resp:	Lungs/O2	DVT Prophylaxis:			
GI: Diet: Last BM:		Skin:	Edema:	Notes:	
GU:			Mobility:		

Assessment   Education   IV's/Lines   Care plan review   I&O's   Chart check
Reassessment   Treatments   Skin   Nursing goals   General care   Sign off

Room:	Name:		Age/Sex:	Admit:

Code:	Allergies:	Isolation:

Attending:	Consults:

Diagnosis:	PMH:

Na:	RBC:	Meds:
K:	WBC:	
Ca:	Hgb:	
Mg:	Hct:	
Ph:	Platelets:	
Cl:	INR:	
Glu:	PTT:	
CO2:	BUN:	
	Creat:	

Diagnostics:	IV:	Fluids:

Vitals:			Intake	Output
T:				
P:				
R:				
BP:				
O2:				

Neuro:	Neuro/CIWA	Cardio/Tele:	Pain Assess:	Pain Reassess:	Blood Sugar:
Resp:	Lungs/O2				
		DVT Prophylaxis:			
GI:					
Diet:					
Last BM:					
GU:		Skin:	Edema:	Notes:	
			Mobility:		

Assessment	Education	IV's/Lines	Care plan review	I&O's	Chart check
Reassessment	Treatments	Skin	Nursing goals	General care	Sign off

Room:	Name:		Age/Sex:	Admit:

Code:	Allergies:	Isolation:

Attending:	Consults:

Diagnosis:	PMH:

Na:	RBC:	Meds:
K:	WBC:	
Ca:	Hgb:	
Mg:	Hct:	
Ph:	Platelets:	
Cl:	INR:	
Glu:	PTT:	
CO2:	BUN:	
	Creat:	

Diagnostics:	IV:	Fluids:

Vitals:			Intake	Output
T:				
P:				
R:				
BP:				
O2:				

Neuro:	Neuro/CIWA	Cardio/Tele:	Pain Assess:	Pain Reassess:	Blood Sugar:
Resp:	Lungs/O2	DVT Prophylaxis:			
GI: Diet: Last BM: GU:		Skin:	Edema: Mobility:	Notes:	

Assessment Education IV's/Lines Care plan review I&O's Chart check
Reassessment Treatments Skin Nursing goals General care Sign off

Room:	Name:		Age/Sex:	Admit:
Code:	Allergies:			Isolation:

Attending:	Consults:
Diagnosis:	PMH:

Na:	RBC:	Meds:
K:	WBC:	
Ca:	Hgb:	
Mg:	Hct:	
Ph:	Platelets:	
Cl:	INR:	
Glu:	PTT:	
CO2:	BUN:	
	Creat:	

Diagnostics:	IV:	Fluids:

Vitals:			Intake	Output
T:				
P:				
R:				
BP:				
O2:				

Neuro:	Neuro/CIWA	Cardio/Tele:	Pain Assess:	Pain Reassess:	Blood Sugar:
Resp:	Lungs/O2				
		DVT Prophylaxis:			
GI:					
Diet:					
Last BM:		Skin:	Edema:	Notes:	
GU:			Mobility:		

Assessment   Education   IV's/Lines   Care plan review   I&O's   Chart check
Reassessment   Treatments   Skin   Nursing goals   General care   Sign off

Room:	Name:		Age/Sex:	Admit:
Code:	Allergies:		Isolation:	

Attending:	Consults:
Diagnosis:	PMH:

Na:	RBC:	Meds:
K:	WBC:	
Ca:	Hgb:	
Mg:	Hct:	
Ph:	Platelets:	
Cl:	INR:	
Glu:	PTT:	
CO2:	BUN:	
	Creat:	

Diagnostics:	IV:	Fluids:

Vitals:			Intake	Output
T:				
P:				
R:				
BP:				
O2:				

Neuro:	Neuro/CIWA	Cardio/Tele:	Pain Assess:	Pain Reassess:	Blood Sugar:
Resp:	Lungs/O2				
		DVT Prophylaxis:			
GI:					
Diet:					
Last BM:		Skin:	Edema:	Notes:	
GU:			Mobility:		

Assessment	Education	IV's/Lines	Care plan review	I&O's	Chart check
Reassessment	Treatments	Skin	Nursing goals	General care	Sign off

Room:	Name:		Age/Sex:	Admit:

Code:	Allergies:	Isolation:

Attending:

Consults:

Diagnosis:

PMH:

Na:	RBC:	Meds:
K:	WBC:	
Ca:	Hgb:	
Mg:	Hct:	
Ph:	Platelets:	
Cl:	INR:	
Glu:	PTT:	
CO2:	BUN:	
	Creat:	

Diagnostics:	IV:	Fluids:

Vitals:			Intake	Output
T:				
P:				
R:				
BP:				
O2:				

Neuro:	Neuro/CIWA	Cardio/Tele:	Pain Assess:	Pain Reassess:	Blood Sugar:
Resp:	Lungs/O2	DVT Prophylaxis:			
GI: Diet: Last BM:		Skin:	Edema:	Notes:	
GU:			Mobility:		

Assessment	Education	IV's/Lines	Care plan review	I&O's	Chart check
Reassessment	Treatments	Skin	Nursing goals	General care	Sign off

Room:	Name:		Age/Sex:	Admit:

Code:	Allergies:		Isolation:

Attending:	Consults:

Diagnosis:	PMH:

Na:	RBC:	Meds:
K:	WBC:	
Ca:	Hgb:	
Mg:	Hct:	
Ph:	Platelets:	
Cl:	INR:	
Glu:	PTT:	
CO2:	BUN:	
	Creat:	

Diagnostics:	IV:	Fluids:

Vitals:			Intake	Output
T:				
P:				
R:				
BP:				
O2:				

Neuro:	Neuro/CIWA	Cardio/Tele:	Pain Assess:	Pain Reassess:	Blood Sugar:
Resp:	Lungs/O2	DVT Prophylaxis:			
GI:					
Diet:					
Last BM:		Skin:	Edema:	Notes:	
GU:			Mobility:		

| Assessment | Education | IV's/Lines | Care plan review | I&O's | Chart check |
| Reassessment | Treatments | Skin | Nursing goals | General care | Sign off |

Room:	Name:		Age/Sex:	Admit:
Code:	Allergies:			Isolation:

Attending:

Consults:

Diagnosis:

PMH:

Na:	RBC:	Meds:
K:	WBC:	
Ca:	Hgb:	
Mg:	Hct:	
Ph:	Platelets:	
Cl:	INR:	
Glu:	PTT:	
CO2:	BUN:	
	Creat:	

Diagnostics:

IV:

Fluids:

Vitals:			Intake	Output
T:				
P:				
R:				
BP:				
O2:				

Neuro:	Neuro/CIWA	Cardio/Tele:	Pain Assess:	Pain Reassess:	Blood Sugar:
Resp:	Lungs/O2	DVT Prophylaxis:			
GI: Diet: Last BM: GU:		Skin:	Edema: Mobility:	Notes:	

| Assessment | Education | IV's/Lines | Care plan review | I&O's | Chart check |
| Reassessment | Treatments | Skin | Nursing goals | General care | Sign off |

Room:	Name:		Age/Sex:	Admit:
Code:	Allergies:			Isolation:

Attending:	Consults:
Diagnosis:	PMH:

Na:	RBC:	Meds:
K:	WBC:	
Ca:	Hgb:	
Mg:	Hct:	
Ph:	Platelets:	
Cl:	INR:	
Glu:	PTT:	
CO2:	BUN:	
	Creat:	

Diagnostics:	IV:	Fluids:

Vitals:			Intake	Output
T:				
P:				
R:				
BP:				
O2:				

Neuro:	Neuro/CIWA	Cardio/Tele:	Pain Assess:	Pain Reassess:	Blood Sugar:
Resp:	Lungs/O2	DVT Prophylaxis:			
GI: Diet: Last BM:		Skin:	Edema:	Notes:	
GU:			Mobility:		

Assessment	Education	IV's/Lines	Care plan review	I&O's	Chart check
Reassessment	Treatments	Skin	Nursing goals	General care	Sign off

Room:	Name:		Age/Sex:	Admit:
Code:	Allergies:			Isolation:

Attending:	Consults:
Diagnosis:	PMH:

Na:	RBC:	Meds:
K:	WBC:	
Ca:	Hgb:	
Mg:	Hct:	
Ph:	Platelets:	
Cl:	INR:	
Glu:	PTT:	
CO2:	BUN:	
	Creat:	

Diagnostics:	IV:	Fluids:

Vitals:			Intake	Output
T:				
P:				
R:				
BP:				
O2:				

Neuro:	Neuro/CIWA	Cardio/Tele:	Pain Assess:	Pain Reassess:	Blood Sugar:
Resp:	Lungs/O2				
		DVT Prophylaxis:			
GI: Diet: Last BM:		Skin:	Edema:	Notes:	
GU:			Mobility:		

Assessment	Education	IV's/Lines	Care plan review	I&O's	Chart check
Reassessment	Treatments	Skin	Nursing goals	General care	Sign off

Room:	Name:		Age/Sex:	Admit:

Code:	Allergies:	Isolation:

Attending:	Consults:

Diagnosis:	PMH:

Na:	RBC:	Meds:
K:	WBC:	
Ca:	Hgb:	
Mg:	Hct:	
Ph:	Platelets:	
Cl:	INR:	
Glu:	PTT:	
CO2:	BUN:	
	Creat:	

Diagnostics:	IV:	Fluids:

Vitals:			Intake	Output
T:				
P:				
R:				
BP:				
O2:				

Neuro:	Neuro/CIWA	Cardio/Tele:	Pain Assess:	Pain Reassess:	Blood Sugar:
Resp:	Lungs/O2	DVT Prophylaxis:			
GI: Diet: Last BM:		Skin:	Edema:	Notes:	
GU:			Mobility:		

Assessment	Education	IV's/Lines	Care plan review	I&O's	Chart check
Reassessment	Treatments	Skin	Nursing goals	General care	Sign off

Room:	Name:		Age/Sex:	Admit:

Code:	Allergies:	Isolation:

Attending:	Consults:

Diagnosis:	PMH:

Na:	RBC:	Meds:
K:	WBC:	
Ca:	Hgb:	
Mg:	Hct:	
Ph:	Platelets:	
Cl:	INR:	
Glu:	PTT:	
CO2:	BUN:	
	Creat:	

Diagnostics:	IV:	Fluids:

Vitals:			Intake	Output
T:				
P:				
R:				
BP:				
O2:				

Neuro:	Neuro/CIWA	Cardio/Tele:	Pain Assess:	Pain Reassess:	Blood Sugar:
Resp:	Lungs/O2				
		DVT Prophylaxis:			
GI:		Skin:	Edema:	Notes:	
Diet:					
Last BM:			Mobility:		
GU:					

Assessment	Education	IV's/Lines	Care plan review	I&O's	Chart check
Reassessment	Treatments	Skin	Nursing goals	General care	Sign off

Room:	Name:		Age/Sex:	Admit:

Code:	Allergies:		Isolation:

Attending:	Consults:

Diagnosis:	PMH:

Na:	RBC:	Meds:
K:	WBC:	
Ca:	Hgb:	
Mg:	Hct:	
Ph:	Platelets:	
Cl:	INR:	
Glu:	PTT:	
CO2:	BUN:	
	Creat:	

Diagnostics:	IV:	Fluids:

Vitals:			Intake	Output
T:				
P:				
R:				
BP:				
O2:				

Neuro:	Neuro/CIWA	Cardio/Tele:	Pain Assess:	Pain Reassess:	Blood Sugar:
Resp:	Lungs/O2				
		DVT Prophylaxis:			
GI: Diet: Last BM:		Skin:	Edema:	Notes:	
GU:			Mobility:		

| Assessment | Education | IV's/Lines | Care plan review | I&O's | Chart check |
| Reassessment | Treatments | Skin | Nursing goals | General care | Sign off |

Room:	Name:		Age/Sex:	Admit:

Code:	Allergies:	Isolation:

Attending:	Consults:

Diagnosis:	PMH:

Na:	RBC:	Meds:
K:	WBC:	
Ca:	Hgb:	
Mg:	Hct:	
Ph:	Platelets:	
Cl:	INR:	
Glu:	PTT:	
CO2:	BUN:	
	Creat:	

Diagnostics:	IV:	Fluids:

Vitals:			Intake	Output
T:				
P:				
R:				
BP:				
O2:				

Neuro:	Neuro/CIWA	Cardio/Tele:	Pain Assess:	Pain Reassess:	Blood Sugar:
Resp:	Lungs/O2	DVT Prophylaxis:			

GI:
  Diet:
  Last BM:
GU:
		Skin:	Edema:
			Mobility:
				Notes:	

Assessment	Education	IV's/Lines	Care plan review	I&O's	Chart check
Reassessment	Treatments	Skin	Nursing goals	General care	Sign off

Room:	Name:		Age/Sex:	Admit:
Code:	Allergies:			Isolation:

Attending:	Consults:
Diagnosis:	PMH:

Na:	RBC:	Meds:
K:	WBC:	
Ca:	Hgb:	
Mg:	Hct:	
Ph:	Platelets:	
Cl:	INR:	
Glu:	PTT:	
CO2:	BUN:	
	Creat:	

Diagnostics:	IV:	Fluids:

Vitals:			Intake	Output
T:				
P:				
R:				
BP:				
O2:				

Neuro:	Neuro/CIWA	Cardio/Tele:	Pain Assess:	Pain Reassess:	Blood Sugar:
Resp:	Lungs/O2	DVT Prophylaxis:			
GI: Diet: Last BM:		Skin:	Edema:	Notes:	
GU:			Mobility:		

Assessment	Education	IV's/Lines	Care plan review	I&O's	Chart check
Reassessment	Treatments	Skin	Nursing goals	General care	Sign off

Room:	Name:		Age/Sex:	Admit:

Code:	Allergies:		Isolation:

Attending:	Consults:

Diagnosis:	PMH:

Na:	RBC:	Meds:
K:	WBC:	
Ca:	Hgb:	
Mg:	Hct:	
Ph:	Platelets:	
Cl:	INR:	
Glu:	PTT:	
CO2:	BUN:	
	Creat:	

Diagnostics:	IV:	Fluids:

Vitals:			Intake	Output
T:				
P:				
R:				
BP:				
O2:				

Neuro:	Neuro/CIWA	Cardio/Tele:	Pain Assess:	Pain Reassess:	Blood Sugar:
Resp:	Lungs/O2	DVT Prophylaxis:			
GI: Diet: Last BM:		Skin:	Edema:	Notes:	
GU:			Mobility:		

Assessment   Education   IV's/Lines   Care plan review   I&O's   Chart check
Reassessment   Treatments   Skin   Nursing goals   General care   Sign off

Room:	Name:		Age/Sex:	Admit:
Code:	Allergies:		Isolation:	

Attending:	Consults:
Diagnosis:	PMH:

Na:	RBC:	Meds:
K:	WBC:	
Ca:	Hgb:	
Mg:	Hct:	
Ph:	Platelets:	
Cl:	INR:	
Glu:	PTT:	
CO2:	BUN:	
	Creat:	

Diagnostics:	IV:	Fluids:

Vitals:			Intake	Output
T:				
P:				
R:				
BP:				
O2:				

Neuro:	Neuro/CIWA	Cardio/Tele:	Pain Assess:	Pain Reassess:	Blood Sugar:
Resp:	Lungs/O2				
		DVT Prophylaxis:			
GI:					
Diet:					
Last BM:		Skin:	Edema:	Notes:	
GU:			Mobility:		

Assessment	Education	IV's/Lines	Care plan review	I&O's	Chart check
Reassessment	Treatments	Skin	Nursing goals	General care	Sign off

Room:	Name:		Age/Sex:	Admit:

Code:	Allergies:		Isolation:

Attending:	Consults:

Diagnosis:	PMH:

Na:	RBC:	Meds:
K:	WBC:	
Ca:	Hgb:	
Mg:	Hct:	
Ph:	Platelets:	
Cl:	INR:	
Glu:	PTT:	
CO2:	BUN:	
	Creat:	

Diagnostics:		IV:	Fluids:

Vitals:			Intake	Output
T:				
P:				
R:				
BP:				
O2:				

Neuro:	Neuro/CIWA	Cardio/Tele:	Pain Assess:	Pain Reassess:	Blood Sugar:
Resp:	Lungs/O2	DVT Prophylaxis:			
GI: Diet: Last BM: GU:		Skin:	Edema: Mobility:	Notes:	

Assessment	Education	IV's/Lines	Care plan review	I&O's	Chart check
Reassessment	Treatments	Skin	Nursing goals	General care	Sign off

Room:	Name:		Age/Sex:	Admit:
Code:	Allergies:			Isolation:

Attending:	Consults:
Diagnosis:	PMH:

Na:	RBC:	Meds:
K:	WBC:	
Ca:	Hgb:	
Mg:	Hct:	
Ph:	Platelets:	
Cl:	INR:	
Glu:	PTT:	
CO2:	BUN:	
	Creat:	

Diagnostics:	IV:	Fluids:

Vitals:			Intake	Output
T:				
P:				
R:				
BP:				
O2:				

Neuro:	Neuro/CIWA	Cardio/Tele:	Pain Assess:	Pain Reassess:	Blood Sugar:
Resp:	Lungs/O2	DVT Prophylaxis:			
GI: Diet: Last BM: GU:		Skin:	Edema: Mobility:	Notes:	

Assessment	Education	IV's/Lines	Care plan review	I&O's	Chart check
Reassessment	Treatments	Skin	Nursing goals	General care	Sign off

Room:	Name:		Age/Sex:	Admit:

Code:	Allergies:	Isolation:

Attending:	Consults:

Diagnosis:	PMH:

Na:	RBC:	Meds:
K:	WBC:	
Ca:	Hgb:	
Mg:	Hct:	
Ph:	Platelets:	
Cl:	INR:	
Glu:	PTT:	
CO2:	BUN:	
	Creat:	

Diagnostics:	IV:	Fluids:

Vitals:			Intake	Output
T:				
P:				
R:				
BP:				
O2:				

Neuro:	Neuro/CIWA	Cardio/Tele:	Pain Assess:	Pain Reassess:	Blood Sugar:
Resp:	Lungs/O2	DVT Prophylaxis:			
GI: Diet: Last BM:					
GU:		Skin:	Edema:	Notes:	
			Mobility:		

Assessment Education IV's/Lines Care plan review I&O's Chart check
Reassessment Treatments Skin Nursing goals General care Sign off

Room:	Name:		Age/Sex:	Admit:
Code:	Allergies:			Isolation:

Attending:

Consults:

Diagnosis:

PMH:

Na:	RBC:	Meds:
K:	WBC:	
Ca:	Hgb:	
Mg:	Hct:	
Ph:	Platelets:	
Cl:	INR:	
Glu:	PTT:	
CO2:	BUN:	
	Creat:	

Diagnostics:	IV:	Fluids:

Vitals:			Intake	Output
T:				
P:				
R:				
BP:				
O2:				

Neuro:	Neuro/CIWA	Cardio/Tele:	Pain Assess:	Pain Reassess:	Blood Sugar:
Resp:	Lungs/O2	DVT Prophylaxis:			
GI: Diet: Last BM: GU:		Skin:	Edema: Mobility:	Notes:	

Assessment	Education	IV's/Lines	Care plan review	I&O's	Chart check
Reassessment	Treatments	Skin	Nursing goals	General care	Sign off

Room:	Name:		Age/Sex:	Admit:
Code:	Allergies:			Isolation:

Attending:

Consults:

Diagnosis:

PMH:

Na:	RBC:	Meds:
K:	WBC:	
Ca:	Hgb:	
Mg:	Hct:	
Ph:	Platelets:	
Cl:	INR:	
Glu:	PTT:	
CO2:	BUN:	
	Creat:	

Diagnostics:	IV:	Fluids:

Vitals:			Intake	Output
T:				
P:				
R:				
BP:				
O2:				

Neuro:	Neuro/CIWA	Cardio/Tele:	Pain Assess:	Pain Reassess:	Blood Sugar:
Resp:	Lungs/O2	DVT Prophylaxis:			
GI: Diet: Last BM: GU:		Skin:	Edema: Mobility:	Notes:	

Assessment	Education	IV's/Lines	Care plan review	I&O's	Chart check
Reassessment	Treatments	Skin	Nursing goals	General care	Sign off

Room:	Name:		Age/Sex:	Admit:
Code:	Allergies:			Isolation:

Attending:	Consults:

Diagnosis:	PMH:

Na:	RBC:	Meds:
K:	WBC:	
Ca:	Hgb:	
Mg:	Hct:	
Ph:	Platelets:	
Cl:	INR:	
Glu:	PTT:	
CO2:	BUN:	
	Creat:	

Diagnostics:	IV:	Fluids:

Vitals:			Intake	Output
T:				
P:				
R:				
BP:				
O2:				

Neuro: Neuro/CIWA	Cardio/Tele:	Pain Assess:	Pain Reassess:	Blood Sugar:
Resp: Lungs/O2	DVT Prophylaxis:			
GI: Diet: Last BM: GU:	Skin:	Edema: Mobility:	Notes:	

Assessment	Education	IV's/Lines	Care plan review	I&O's	Chart check
Reassessment	Treatments	Skin	Nursing goals	General care	Sign off

Room:	Name:		Age/Sex:	Admit:

Code:	Allergies:	Isolation:

Attending:	Consults:

Diagnosis:	PMH:

Na:	RBC:	Meds:
K:	WBC:	
Ca:	Hgb:	
Mg:	Hct:	
Ph:	Platelets:	
Cl:	INR:	
Glu:	PTT:	
CO2:	BUN:	
	Creat:	

Diagnostics:	IV:	Fluids:

Vitals:			Intake	Output
T:				
P:				
R:				
BP:				
O2:				

Neuro:	Neuro/CIWA	Cardio/Tele:	Pain Assess:	Pain Reassess:	Blood Sugar:
Resp:	Lungs/O2				
		DVT Prophylaxis:			
GI: Diet: Last BM:		Skin:	Edema:	Notes:	
GU:			Mobility:		

Assessment	Education	IV's/Lines	Care plan review	I&O's	Chart check
Reassessment	Treatments	Skin	Nursing goals	General care	Sign off

Room:	Name:		Age/Sex:	Admit:

Code:	Allergies:		Isolation:

Attending:	Consults:

Diagnosis:	PMH:

Na:	RBC:	Meds:
K:	WBC:	
Ca:	Hgb:	
Mg:	Hct:	
Ph:	Platelets:	
Cl:	INR:	
Glu:	PTT:	
CO2:	BUN:	
	Creat:	

Diagnostics:	IV:	Fluids:

Vitals:			Intake	Output
T:				
P:				
R:				
BP:				
O2:				

Neuro:	Neuro/CIWA	Cardio/Tele:	Pain Assess:	Pain Reassess:	Blood Sugar:
Resp:	Lungs/O2	DVT Prophylaxis:			
GI: Diet: Last BM:		Skin:	Edema:	Notes:	
GU:			Mobility:		

Assessment	Education	IV's/Lines	Care plan review	I&O's	Chart check
Reassessment	Treatments	Skin	Nursing goals	General care	Sign off

Room:	Name:		Age/Sex:	Admit:
Code:	Allergies:			Isolation:

Attending:	Consults:
Diagnosis:	PMH:

Na:	RBC:	Meds:
K:	WBC:	
Ca:	Hgb:	
Mg:	Hct:	
Ph:	Platelets:	
Cl:	INR:	
Glu:	PTT:	
CO2:	BUN:	
	Creat:	

Diagnostics:	IV:	Fluids:

Vitals:			Intake	Output
T:				
P:				
R:				
BP:				
O2:				

Neuro:	Neuro/CIWA	Cardio/Tele:	Pain Assess:	Pain Reassess:	Blood Sugar:
Resp:	Lungs/O2	DVT Prophylaxis:			
GI: Diet: Last BM:		Skin:	Edema:	Notes:	
GU:			Mobility:		

Assessment	Education	IV's/Lines	Care plan review	I&O's	Chart check
Reassessment	Treatments	Skin	Nursing goals	General care	Sign off

Room:	Name:		Age/Sex:	Admit:

Code:	Allergies:		Isolation:

Attending:	Consults:

Diagnosis:	PMH:

Na:	RBC:	Meds:
K:	WBC:	
Ca:	Hgb:	
Mg:	Hct:	
Ph:	Platelets:	
Cl:	INR:	
Glu:	PTT:	
CO2:	BUN:	
	Creat:	

Diagnostics:	IV:	Fluids:

Vitals:			Intake	Output
T:				
P:				
R:				
BP:				
O2:				

Neuro:	Neuro/CIWA	Cardio/Tele:	Pain Assess:	Pain Reassess:	Blood Sugar:
Resp:	Lungs/O2	DVT Prophylaxis:			
GI: Diet: Last BM:		Skin:	Edema:	Notes:	
GU:			Mobility:		

Assessment   Education   IV's/Lines   Care plan review   I&O's   Chart check

Reassessment   Treatments   Skin   Nursing goals   General care   Sign off

Room:	Name:		Age/Sex:	Admit:

Code:	Allergies:	Isolation:

Attending:

Consults:

Diagnosis:

PMH:

Na:	RBC:	Meds:
K:	WBC:	
Ca:	Hgb:	
Mg:	Hct:	
Ph:	Platelets:	
Cl:	INR:	
Glu:	PTT:	
CO2:	BUN:	
	Creat:	

Diagnostics:

IV:

Fluids:

Vitals:			Intake	Output
T:				
P:				
R:				
BP:				
O2:				

Neuro:	Neuro/CIWA	Cardio/Tele:	Pain Assess:	Pain Reassess:	Blood Sugar:
Resp:	Lungs/O2	DVT Prophylaxis:			
GI: Diet: Last BM:		Skin:	Edema:	Notes:	
GU:			Mobility:		

Assessment	Education	IV's/Lines	Care plan review	I&O's	Chart check
Reassessment	Treatments	Skin	Nursing goals	General care	Sign off

Room:	Name:		Age/Sex:	Admit:
Code:	Allergies:		Isolation:	

Attending:	Consults:
Diagnosis:	PMH:

Na:	RBC:	Meds:
K:	WBC:	
Ca:	Hgb:	
Mg:	Hct:	
Ph:	Platelets:	
Cl:	INR:	
Glu:	PTT:	
CO2:	BUN:	
	Creat:	

Diagnostics:	IV:	Fluids:

Vitals:			Intake	Output
T:				
P:				
R:				
BP:				
O2:				

Neuro:	Neuro/CIWA	Cardio/Tele:	Pain Assess:	Pain Reassess:	Blood Sugar:
Resp:	Lungs/O2	DVT Prophylaxis:			

GI:
  Diet:
  Last BM:
GU:
		Skin:	Edema:
			Mobility:
				Notes:	

Assessment	Education	IV's/Lines	Care plan review	I&O's	Chart check
Reassessment	Treatments	Skin	Nursing goals	General care	Sign off

Room:	Name:			Age/Sex:	Admit:
Code:	Allergies:				Isolation:

Attending:	Consults:
Diagnosis:	PMH:

Na:	RBC:	Meds:
K:	WBC:	
Ca:	Hgb:	
Mg:	Hct:	
Ph:	Platelets:	
Cl:	INR:	
Glu:	PTT:	
CO2:	BUN:	
	Creat:	

Diagnostics:	IV:	Fluids:

Vitals:			Intake	Output
T:				
P:				
R:				
BP:				
O2:				

Neuro:	Neuro/CIWA	Cardio/Tele:	Pain Assess:	Pain Reassess:	Blood Sugar:
Resp:	Lungs/O2				
		DVT Prophylaxis:			
GI:					
Diet:		Skin:	Edema:	Notes:	
Last BM:			Mobility:		
GU:					

Assessment   Education   IV's/Lines   Care plan review   I&O's   Chart check
Reassessment   Treatments   Skin   Nursing goals   General care   Sign off

Room:	Name:		Age/Sex:	Admit:
Code:	Allergies:			Isolation:

Attending:

Consults:

Diagnosis:

PMH:

Na:	RBC:	Meds:
K:	WBC:	
Ca:	Hgb:	
Mg:	Hct:	
Ph:	Platelets:	
Cl:	INR:	
Glu:	PTT:	
CO2:	BUN:	
	Creat:	

Diagnostics:	IV:	Fluids:

Vitals:			Intake	Output
T:				
P:				
R:				
BP:				
O2:				

Neuro:	Neuro/CIWA	Cardio/Tele:	Pain Assess:	Pain Reassess:	Blood Sugar:
Resp:	Lungs/O2	DVT Prophylaxis:			
GI: Diet: Last BM:		Skin:	Edema:	Notes:	
GU:			Mobility:		

Assessment	Education	IV's/Lines	Care plan review	I&O's	Chart check
Reassessment	Treatments	Skin	Nursing goals	General care	Sign off

Room:	Name:		Age/Sex:	Admit:

Code:	Allergies:	Isolation:

Attending:	Consults:

Diagnosis:	PMH:

Na:	RBC:	Meds:
K:	WBC:	
Ca:	Hgb:	
Mg:	Hct:	
Ph:	Platelets:	
Cl:	INR:	
Glu:	PTT:	
CO2:	BUN:	
	Creat:	

Diagnostics:	IV:	Fluids:

Vitals:			Intake	Output
T:				
P:				
R:				
BP:				
O2:				

Neuro:	Neuro/CIWA	Cardio/Tele:	Pain Assess:	Pain Reassess:	Blood Sugar:
Resp:	Lungs/O2	DVT Prophylaxis:			
GI: Diet: Last BM: GU:		Skin:	Edema: Mobility:	Notes:	

Assessment	Education	IV's/Lines	Care plan review	I&O's	Chart check
Reassessment	Treatments	Skin	Nursing goals	General care	Sign off

Room:	Name:		Age/Sex:	Admit:
Code:	Allergies:		Isolation:	

Attending:	Consults:
Diagnosis:	PMH:

Na:	RBC:	Meds:
K:	WBC:	
Ca:	Hgb:	
Mg:	Hct:	
Ph:	Platelets:	
Cl:	INR:	
Glu:	PTT:	
CO2:	BUN:	
	Creat:	

Diagnostics:	IV:	Fluids:

Vitals:			Intake	Output
T:				
P:				
R:				
BP:				
O2:				

Neuro:	Neuro/CIWA	Cardio/Tele:	Pain Assess:	Pain Reassess:	Blood Sugar:
Resp:	Lungs/O2	DVT Prophylaxis:			
GI: Diet: Last BM:		Skin:	Edema: Mobility:	Notes:	
GU:					

Assessment	Education	IV's/Lines	Care plan review	I&O's	Chart check
Reassessment	Treatments	Skin	Nursing goals	General care	Sign off

Room:	Name:		Age/Sex:	Admit:
Code:	Allergies:			Isolation:

Attending:	Consults:
Diagnosis:	PMH:

Na:	RBC:	Meds:
K:	WBC:	
Ca:	Hgb:	
Mg:	Hct:	
Ph:	Platelets:	
Cl:	INR:	
Glu:	PTT:	
CO2:	BUN:	
	Creat:	

Diagnostics:	IV:	Fluids:

Vitals:			Intake	Output
T:				
P:				
R:				
BP:				
O2:				

Neuro:	Neuro/CIWA	Cardio/Tele:	Pain Assess:	Pain Reassess:	Blood Sugar:
Resp:	Lungs/O2	DVT Prophylaxis:			
GI: Diet: Last BM:		Skin:	Edema:	Notes:	
GU:			Mobility:		

| Assessment | Education | IV's/Lines | Care plan review | I&O's | Chart check |
| Reassessment | Treatments | Skin | Nursing goals | General care | Sign off |

Room:	Name:		Age/Sex:	Admit:

Code:	Allergies:		Isolation:

Attending:	Consults:

Diagnosis:	PMH:

Na:	RBC:	Meds:
K:	WBC:	
Ca:	Hgb:	
Mg:	Hct:	
Ph:	Platelets:	
Cl:	INR:	
Glu:	PTT:	
CO2:	BUN:	
	Creat:	

Diagnostics:	IV:	Fluids:

Vitals:			Intake	Output
T:				
P:				
R:				
BP:				
O2:				

Neuro:	Neuro/CIWA	Cardio/Tele:	Pain Assess:	Pain Reassess:	Blood Sugar:
Resp:	Lungs/O2	DVT Prophylaxis:			
GI: Diet: Last BM: GU:		Skin:	Edema: Mobility:	Notes:	

Assessment   Education   IV's/Lines   Care plan review   I&O's   Chart check
Reassessment   Treatments   Skin   Nursing goals   General care   Sign off

Room:	Name:		Age/Sex:	Admit:
Code:	Allergies:			Isolation:

Attending:	Consults:
Diagnosis:	PMH:

Na:	RBC:	Meds:
K:	WBC:	
Ca:	Hgb:	
Mg:	Hct:	
Ph:	Platelets:	
Cl:	INR:	
Glu:	PTT:	
CO2:	BUN:	
	Creat:	

Diagnostics:	IV:	Fluids:

Vitals:			Intake	Output
T:				
P:				
R:				
BP:				
O2:				

Neuro:	Neuro/CIWA	Cardio/Tele:	Pain Assess:	Pain Reassess:	Blood Sugar:
Resp:	Lungs/O2				
		DVT Prophylaxis:			
GI: Diet: Last BM:		Skin:	Edema:	Notes:	
GU:			Mobility:		

Assessment	Education	IV's/Lines	Care plan review	I&O's	Chart check
Reassessment	Treatments	Skin	Nursing goals	General care	Sign off

Room:	Name:		Age/Sex:	Admit:
Code:	Allergies:		Isolation:	

Attending:	Consults:
Diagnosis:	PMH:

Na:	RBC:	Meds:
K:	WBC:	
Ca:	Hgb:	
Mg:	Hct:	
Ph:	Platelets:	
Cl:	INR:	
Glu:	PTT:	
CO2:	BUN:	
	Creat:	

Diagnostics:	IV:	Fluids:

Vitals:			Intake	Output
T:				
P:				
R:				
BP:				
O2:				

Neuro:	Neuro/CIWA	Cardio/Tele:	Pain Assess:	Pain Reassess:	Blood Sugar:
Resp:	Lungs/O2	DVT Prophylaxis:			
GI: Diet: Last BM:		Skin:	Edema:	Notes:	
GU:			Mobility:		

Assessment	Education	IV's/Lines	Care plan review	I&O's	Chart check
Reassessment	Treatments	Skin	Nursing goals	General care	Sign off

Room:	Name:		Age/Sex:	Admit:

Code:	Allergies:	Isolation:

Attending: | **Consults:**

Diagnosis: | **PMH:**

Na:	RBC:	Meds:
K:	WBC:	
Ca:	Hgb:	
Mg:	Hct:	
Ph:	Platelets:	
Cl:	INR:	
Glu:	PTT:	
CO2:	BUN:	
	Creat:	

Diagnostics:	IV:	Fluids:

Vitals:			Intake	Output
T:				
P:				
R:				
BP:				
O2:				

Neuro:	Neuro/CIWA	Cardio/Tele:	Pain Assess:	Pain Reassess:	Blood Sugar:
Resp:	Lungs/O2	DVT Prophylaxis:			

GI:
  Diet:
  Last BM:
 	
GU:
		Skin:	Edema:	Notes:	

			Mobility:		

Assessment	Education	IV's/Lines	Care plan review	I&O's	Chart check
Reassessment	Treatments	Skin	Nursing goals	General care	Sign off

Room:	Name:		Age/Sex:	Admit:
Code:	Allergies:			Isolation:

Attending:	Consults:
Diagnosis:	PMH:

Na:	RBC:	Meds:
K:	WBC:	
Ca:	Hgb:	
Mg:	Hct:	
Ph:	Platelets:	
Cl:	INR:	
Glu:	PTT:	
CO2:	BUN:	
	Creat:	

Diagnostics:	IV:	Fluids:

Vitals:			Intake	Output
T:				
P:				
R:				
BP:				
O2:				

Neuro:	Neuro/CIWA	Cardio/Tele:	Pain Assess:	Pain Reassess:	Blood Sugar:
Resp:	Lungs/O2	DVT Prophylaxis:			
GI: Diet: Last BM: GU:		Skin:	Edema: Mobility:	Notes:	

| Assessment | Education | IV's/Lines | Care plan review | I&O's | Chart check |
| Reassessment | Treatments | Skin | Nursing goals | General care | Sign off |

| Room: | Name: | | Age/Sex: | Admit: |

| Code: | Allergies: | Isolation: |

| Attending: | Consults: |

| Diagnosis: | PMH: |

Na:	RBC:	Meds:
K:	WBC:	
Ca:	Hgb:	
Mg:	Hct:	
Ph:	Platelets:	
Cl:	INR:	
Glu:	PTT:	
CO_2:	BUN:	
	Creat:	

| Diagnostics: | IV: | Fluids: |

Vitals:			Intake	Output
T:				
P:				
R:				
BP:				
O2:				

Neuro:	Neuro/CIWA	Cardio/Tele:	Pain Assess:	Pain Reassess:	Blood Sugar:
Resp:	Lungs/O2				
		DVT Prophylaxis:			
GI:					
Diet:					
Last BM:		Skin:	Edema:	Notes:	
GU:			Mobility:		

Assessment   Education   IV's/Lines   Care plan review   I&O's   Chart check
Reassessment   Treatments   Skin   Nursing goals   General care   Sign off

Room:	Name:		Age/Sex:	Admit:
Code:	Allergies:			Isolation:

Attending:	Consults:
Diagnosis:	PMH:

Na:	RBC:	Meds:
K:	WBC:	
Ca:	Hgb:	
Mg:	Hct:	
Ph:	Platelets:	
Cl:	INR:	
Glu:	PTT:	
CO2:	BUN:	
	Creat:	

Diagnostics:	IV:	Fluids:

Vitals:			Intake	Output
T:				
P:				
R:				
BP:				
O2:				

Neuro:	Neuro/CIWA	Cardio/Tele:	Pain Assess:	Pain Reassess:	Blood Sugar:
Resp:	Lungs/O2	DVT Prophylaxis:			
GI: Diet: Last BM:		Skin:	Edema:	Notes:	
GU:			Mobility:		

Assessment	Education	IV's/Lines	Care plan review	I&O's	Chart check
Reassessment	Treatments	Skin	Nursing goals	General care	Sign off

Room:	Name:		Age/Sex:	Admit:
Code:	Allergies:			Isolation:

Attending:	Consults:
Diagnosis:	PMH:

Na:	RBC:	Meds:
K:	WBC:	
Ca:	Hgb:	
Mg:	Hct:	
Ph:	Platelets:	
Cl:	INR:	
Glu:	PTT:	
CO2:	BUN:	
	Creat:	

Diagnostics:	IV:	Fluids:

Vitals:			Intake	Output
T:				
P:				
R:				
BP:				
O2:				

Neuro:	Neuro/CIWA	Cardio/Tele:	Pain Assess:	Pain Reassess:	Blood Sugar:
Resp:	Lungs/O2	DVT Prophylaxis:			
GI: Diet: Last BM:					
GU:		Skin:	Edema: Mobility:	Notes:	

Assessment   Education   IV's/Lines   Care plan review   I&O's   Chart check
Reassessment   Treatments   Skin   Nursing goals   General care   Sign off

Room:	Name:		Age/Sex:	Admit:

Code:	Allergies:			Isolation:

Attending:	Consults:

Diagnosis:	PMH:

Na:	RBC:	Meds:
K:	WBC:	
Ca:	Hgb:	
Mg:	Hct:	
Ph:	Platelets:	
Cl:	INR:	
Glu:	PTT:	
CO2:	BUN:	
	Creat:	

Diagnostics:	IV:	Fluids:

Vitals:			Intake	Output
T:				
P:				
R:				
BP:				
O2:				

Neuro:	Neuro/CIWA	Cardio/Tele:	Pain Assess:	Pain Reassess:	Blood Sugar:
Resp:	Lungs/O2	DVT Prophylaxis:			
GI: Diet: Last BM: GU:		Skin:	Edema: Mobility:	Notes:	

Assessment   Education   IV's/Lines   Care plan review   I&O's   Chart check
Reassessment   Treatments   Skin   Nursing goals   General care Sign off

Room:	Name:		Age/Sex:	Admit:

Code:	Allergies:		Isolation:

Attending:	Consults:

Diagnosis:	PMH:

Na:	RBC:	Meds:
K:	WBC:	
Ca:	Hgb:	
Mg:	Hct:	
Ph:	Platelets:	
Cl:	INR:	
Glu:	PTT:	
CO2:	BUN:	
	Creat:	

Diagnostics:	IV:	Fluids:

Vitals:			Intake	Output
T:				
P:				
R:				
BP:				
O2:				

Neuro:	Neuro/CIWA	Cardio/Tele:	Pain Assess:	Pain Reassess:	Blood Sugar:
Resp:	Lungs/O2	DVT Prophylaxis:			
GI: Diet: Last BM: GU:		Skin:	Edema:	Notes:	
			Mobility:		

Assessment	Education	IV's/Lines	Care plan review	I&O's	Chart check
Reassessment	Treatments	Skin	Nursing goals	General care	Sign off

Room:	Name:		Age/Sex:	Admit:
Code:	Allergies:			Isolation:

Attending:	Consults:
Diagnosis:	PMH:

Na:	RBC:	Meds:
K:	WBC:	
Ca:	Hgb:	
Mg:	Hct:	
Ph:	Platelets:	
Cl:	INR:	
Glu:	PTT:	
CO2:	BUN:	
	Creat:	

Diagnostics:		IV:	Fluids:

Vitals:			Intake	Output
T:				
P:				
R:				
BP:				
O2:				

Neuro:	Neuro/CIWA	Cardio/Tele:	Pain Assess:	Pain Reassess:	Blood Sugar:
Resp:	Lungs/O2	DVT Prophylaxis:			
GI:
Diet:
Last BM:		Skin:	Edema:	Notes:	
GU:			Mobility:		

Assessment	Education	IV's/Lines	Care plan review	I&O's	Chart check
Reassessment	Treatments	Skin	Nursing goals	General care	Sign off

Room:	Name:		Age/Sex:	Admit:
Code:	Allergies:			Isolation:

Attending:

Consults:

Diagnosis:

PMH:

		Meds:
Na:	RBC:	
K:	WBC:	
Ca:	Hgb:	
Mg:	Hct:	
Ph:	Platelets:	
Cl:	INR:	
Glu:	PTT:	
CO2:	BUN:	
	Creat:	

Diagnostics:	IV:	Fluids:

Vitals:			Intake	Output
T:				
P:				
R:				
BP:				
O2:				

Neuro:	Neuro/CIWA	Cardio/Tele:	Pain Assess:	Pain Reassess:	Blood Sugar:
Resp:	Lungs/O2	DVT Prophylaxis:			
GI: Diet: Last BM:					
GU:		Skin:	Edema:	Notes:	
			Mobility:		

| Assessment | Education | IV's/Lines | Care plan review | I&O's | Chart check |
| Reassessment | Treatments | Skin | Nursing goals | General care | Sign off |

Room:	Name:		Age/Sex:	Admit:
Code:	Allergies:			Isolation:

Attending:	Consults:

Diagnosis:	PMH:

Na:	RBC:	Meds:
K:	WBC:	
Ca:	Hgb:	
Mg:	Hct:	
Ph:	Platelets:	
Cl:	INR:	
Glu:	PTT:	
CO2:	BUN:	
	Creat:	

Diagnostics:	IV:	Fluids:

Vitals:			Intake	Output
T:				
P:				
R:				
BP:				
O2:				

Neuro:	Neuro/CIWA	Cardio/Tele:	Pain Assess:	Pain Reassess:	Blood Sugar:
Resp:	Lungs/O2	DVT Prophylaxis:			

GI:
  Diet:
  Last BM:
 	
GU:
		Skin:	Edema:
			
			Mobility:
				Notes:	

Assessment	Education	IV's/Lines	Care plan review	I&O's	Chart check
Reassessment	Treatments	Skin	Nursing goals	General care	Sign off

Room:	Name:		Age/Sex:	Admit:

Code:	Allergies:	Isolation:

Attending:	Consults:

Diagnosis:	PMH:

Na:	RBC:	Meds:
K:	WBC:	
Ca:	Hgb:	
Mg:	Hct:	
Ph:	Platelets:	
Cl:	INR:	
Glu:	PTT:	
CO2:	BUN:	
	Creat:	

Diagnostics:	IV:	Fluids:

Vitals:			Intake	Output
T:				
P:				
R:				
BP:				
O2:				

Neuro:	Neuro/CIWA	Cardio/Tele:	Pain Assess:	Pain Reassess:	Blood Sugar:
Resp:	Lungs/O2	DVT Prophylaxis:			
GI: Diet: Last BM:		Skin:	Edema:	Notes:	
GU:			Mobility:		

Assessment	Education	IV's/Lines	Care plan review	I&O's	Chart check
Reassessment	Treatments	Skin	Nursing goals	General care	Sign off

Room:	Name:		Age/Sex:	Admit:

Code:	Allergies:	Isolation:

Attending:	Consults:

Diagnosis:	PMH:

Na:	RBC:	Meds:
K:	WBC:	
Ca:	Hgb:	
Mg:	Hct:	
Ph:	Platelets:	
Cl:	INR:	
Glu:	PTT:	
CO2:	BUN:	
	Creat:	

Diagnostics:	IV:	Fluids:

Vitals:			Intake	Output
T:				
P:				
R:				
BP:				
O2:				

Neuro:	Neuro/CIWA	Cardio/Tele:	Pain Assess:	Pain Reassess:	Blood Sugar:
Resp:	Lungs/O2				
		DVT Prophylaxis:			

GI:
  Diet:
  Last BM:
 	
GU:
		Skin:	Edema:
			
			Mobility:
				Notes:	

Assessment　　　Education　　　IV's/Lines　　　Care plan review　　　I&O's　　　Chart check
Reassessment　　　Treatments　　　Skin　　　Nursing goals　　　General care　　　Sign off

Room:	Name:		Age/Sex:	Admit:

Code:	Allergies:	Isolation:

Attending:

Consults:

Diagnosis:

PMH:

Na:	RBC:	Meds:
K:	WBC:	
Ca:	Hgb:	
Mg:	Hct:	
Ph:	Platelets:	
Cl:	INR:	
Glu:	PTT:	
CO2:	BUN:	
	Creat:	

Diagnostics:	IV:	Fluids:

Vitals:			Intake	Output
T:				
P:				
R:				
BP:				
O2:				

Neuro: Neuro/CIWA	Cardio/Tele:	Pain Assess:	Pain Reassess:	Blood Sugar:
Resp: Lungs/O2	DVT Prophylaxis:			
GI: Diet: Last BM: GU:	Skin:	Edema: Mobility:	Notes:	

| Assessment | Education | IV's/Lines | Care plan review | I&O's | Chart check |
| Reassessment | Treatments | Skin | Nursing goals | General care | Sign off |

Room:	Name:		Age/Sex:	Admit:
Code:	Allergies:			Isolation:

Attending:

Consults:

Diagnosis:

PMH:

Na:	RBC:	Meds:
K:	WBC:	
Ca:	Hgb:	
Mg:	Hct:	
Ph:	Platelets:	
Cl:	INR:	
Glu:	PTT:	
CO2:	BUN:	
	Creat:	

Diagnostics:	IV:	Fluids:

Vitals:			Intake	Output
T:				
P:				
R:				
BP:				
O2:				

Neuro:	Neuro/CIWA	Cardio/Tele:	Pain Assess:	Pain Reassess:	Blood Sugar:
Resp:	Lungs/O2	DVT Prophylaxis:			
GI: Diet: Last BM:		Skin:	Edema:	Notes:	
GU:			Mobility:		

Assessment	Education	IV's/Lines	Care plan review	I&O's	Chart check
Reassessment	Treatments	Skin	Nursing goals	General care	Sign off

Room:	Name:		Age/Sex:	Admit:

Code:	Allergies:	Isolation:

Attending:	Consults:

Diagnosis:	PMH:

Na:	RBC:	Meds:
K:	WBC:	
Ca:	Hgb:	
Mg:	Hct:	
Ph:	Platelets:	
Cl:	INR:	
Glu:	PTT:	
CO2:	BUN:	
	Creat:	

Diagnostics:	IV:	Fluids:

Vitals:			Intake	Output
T:				
P:				
R:				
BP:				
O2:				

Neuro:	Neuro/CIWA	Cardio/Tele:	Pain Assess:	Pain Reassess:	Blood Sugar:
Resp:	Lungs/O2	DVT Prophylaxis:			
GI: Diet: Last BM:		Skin:	Edema:	Notes:	
GU:			Mobility:		

Assessment	Education	IV's/Lines	Care plan review	I&O's	Chart check
Reassessment	Treatments	Skin	Nursing goals	General care	Sign off

Room:	Name:		Age/Sex:	Admit:

Code:	Allergies:	Isolation:

Attending:	Consults:

Diagnosis:	PMH:

Na:	RBC:	Meds:
K:	WBC:	
Ca:	Hgb:	
Mg:	Hct:	
Ph:	Platelets:	
Cl:	INR:	
Glu:	PTT:	
CO2:	BUN:	
	Creat:	

Diagnostics:	IV:	Fluids:

Vitals:			Intake	Output
T:				
P:				
R:				
BP:				
O2:				

Neuro:	Neuro/CIWA	Cardio/Tele:	Pain Assess:	Pain Reassess:	Blood Sugar:
Resp:	Lungs/O2	DVT Prophylaxis:			
GI: Diet: Last BM: GU:		Skin:	Edema: Mobility:	Notes:	

Assessment	Education	IV's/Lines	Care plan review	I&O's	Chart check
Reassessment	Treatments	Skin	Nursing goals	General care	Sign off

Room:	Name:		Age/Sex:	Admit:

Code:	Allergies:	Isolation:

Attending:	Consults:

Diagnosis:	PMH:

Na:	RBC:	Meds:
K:	WBC:	
Ca:	Hgb:	
Mg:	Hct:	
Ph:	Platelets:	
Cl:	INR:	
Glu:	PTT:	
CO2:	BUN:	
	Creat:	

Diagnostics:	IV:	Fluids:

Vitals:			Intake	Output
T:				
P:				
R:				
BP:				
O2:				

Neuro:	Neuro/CIWA	Cardio/Tele:	Pain Assess:	Pain Reassess:	Blood Sugar:
Resp:	Lungs/O2	DVT Prophylaxis:			
GI: Diet: Last BM: GU:		Skin:	Edema: Mobility:	Notes:	

Assessment   Education   IV's/Lines   Care plan review   I&O's   Chart check
Reassessment   Treatments   Skin   Nursing goals   General care   Sign off

Room:	Name:		Age/Sex:	Admit:
Code:	Allergies:			Isolation:

Attending:

Consults:

Diagnosis:

PMH:

Na:	RBC:	Meds:
K:	WBC:	
Ca:	Hgb:	
Mg:	Hct:	
Ph:	Platelets:	
Cl:	INR:	
Glu:	PTT:	
CO2:	BUN:	
	Creat:	

Diagnostics:	IV:	Fluids:

Vitals:			Intake	Output
T:				
P:				
R:				
BP:				
O2:				

Neuro:	Neuro/CIWA	Cardio/Tele:	Pain Assess:	Pain Reassess:	Blood Sugar:
Resp:	Lungs/O2	DVT Prophylaxis:			
GI: Diet: Last BM:		Skin:	Edema:	Notes:	
GU:			Mobility:		

Assessment	Education	IV's/Lines	Care plan review	I&O's	Chart check
Reassessment	Treatments	Skin	Nursing goals	General care	Sign off

Room:	Name:		Age/Sex:	Admit:

Code:	Allergies:	Isolation:

Attending:

Consults:

Diagnosis:

PMH:

Na:	RBC:	**Meds:**
K:	WBC:	
Ca:	Hgb:	
Mg:	Hct:	
Ph:	Platelets:	
Cl:	INR:	
Glu:	PTT:	
CO2:	BUN:	
	Creat:	

Diagnostics:	IV:	Fluids:

Vitals:			Intake	Output
T:				
P:				
R:				
BP:				
O2:				

Neuro:	Neuro/CIWA	Cardio/Tele:	Pain Assess:	Pain Reassess:	Blood Sugar:
Resp:	Lungs/O2				
		DVT Prophylaxis:			
GI:					
Diet:		Skin:	Edema:	Notes:	
Last BM:					
GU:			Mobility:		

Assessment	Education	IV's/Lines	Care plan review	I&O's	Chart check
Reassessment	Treatments	Skin	Nursing goals	General care	Sign off

Room:	Name:		Age/Sex:	Admit:

Code:	Allergies:		Isolation:

Attending:	Consults:

Diagnosis:	PMH:

Na:	RBC:	Meds:
K:	WBC:	
Ca:	Hgb:	
Mg:	Hct:	
Ph:	Platelets:	
Cl:	INR:	
Glu:	PTT:	
CO_2:	BUN:	
	Creat:	

Diagnostics:	IV:	Fluids:

Vitals:			Intake	Output
T:				
P:				
R:				
BP:				
O2:				

Neuro:	Neuro/CIWA	Cardio/Tele:	Pain Assess:	Pain Reassess:	Blood Sugar:
Resp:	Lungs/O2	DVT Prophylaxis:			
GI: Diet: Last BM: GU:		Skin:	Edema: Mobility:	Notes:	

Assessment   Education   IV's/Lines   Care plan review   I&O's   Chart check
Reassessment   Treatments   Skin   Nursing goals   General care   Sign off

Room:	Name:		Age/Sex:	Admit:
Code:	Allergies:			Isolation:

Attending:	Consults:
Diagnosis:	PMH:

Na:	RBC:	Meds:
K:	WBC:	
Ca:	Hgb:	
Mg:	Hct:	
Ph:	Platelets:	
Cl:	INR:	
Glu:	PTT:	
CO2:	BUN:	
	Creat:	

Diagnostics:	IV:	Fluids:

Vitals:			Intake	Output
T:				
P:				
R:				
BP:				
O2:				

Neuro:	Neuro/CIWA	Cardio/Tele:	Pain Assess:	Pain Reassess:	Blood Sugar:
Resp:	Lungs/O2	DVT Prophylaxis:			
GI: Diet: Last BM:		Skin:	Edema:	Notes:	
GU:			Mobility:		

Assessment	Education	IV's/Lines	Care plan review	I&O's	Chart check
Reassessment	Treatments	Skin	Nursing goals	General care	Sign off

Room:	Name:		Age/Sex:	Admit:

Code:	Allergies:		Isolation:

Attending:	Consults:

Diagnosis:	PMH:

Na:	RBC:	Meds:
K:	WBC:	
Ca:	Hgb:	
Mg:	Hct:	
Ph:	Platelets:	
Cl:	INR:	
Glu:	PTT:	
CO_2:	BUN:	
	Creat:	

Diagnostics:	IV:	Fluids:

Vitals:			Intake	Output
T:				
P:				
R:				
BP:				
O2:				

Neuro:	Neuro/CIWA	Cardio/Tele:	Pain Assess:	Pain Reassess:	Blood Sugar:
Resp:	Lungs/O2	DVT Prophylaxis:			
GI: Diet: Last BM:		Skin:	Edema:	Notes:	
GU:			Mobility:		

Assessment	Education	IV's/Lines	Care plan review	I&O's	Chart check
Reassessment	Treatments	Skin	Nursing goals	General care	Sign off

Room:	Name:		Age/Sex:	Admit:

Code:	Allergies:		Isolation:

Attending:	Consults:

Diagnosis:	PMH:

Na:	RBC:	Meds:
K:	WBC:	
Ca:	Hgb:	
Mg:	Hct:	
Ph:	Platelets:	
Cl:	INR:	
Glu:	PTT:	
CO2:	BUN:	
	Creat:	

Diagnostics:	IV:	Fluids:

Vitals:			Intake	Output
T:				
P:				
R:				
BP:				
O2:				

Neuro:	Neuro/CIWA	Cardio/Tele:	Pain Assess:	Pain Reassess:	Blood Sugar:
Resp:	Lungs/O2				
		DVT Prophylaxis:			
GI:					
Diet:					
Last BM:		Skin:	Edema:	Notes:	
GU:			Mobility:		

Assessment	Education	IV's/Lines	Care plan review	I&O's	Chart check
Reassessment	Treatments	Skin	Nursing goals	General care	Sign off

Room:	Name:		Age/Sex:	Admit:

Code:	Allergies:		Isolation:

Attending:	Consults:

Diagnosis:	PMH:

Na:	RBC:	Meds:
K:	WBC:	
Ca:	Hgb:	
Mg:	Hct:	
Ph:	Platelets:	
Cl:	INR:	
Glu:	PTT:	
CO2:	BUN:	
	Creat:	

Diagnostics:	IV:	Fluids:

Vitals:			Intake	Output
T:				
P:				
R:				
BP:				
O2:				

Neuro: Neuro/CIWA	Cardio/Tele:	Pain Assess:	Pain Reassess:	Blood Sugar:
Resp: Lungs/O2	DVT Prophylaxis:			
GI: Diet: Last BM:	Skin:	Edema:	Notes:	
GU:		Mobility:		

Assessment	Education	IV's/Lines	Care plan review	I&O's	Chart check
Reassessment	Treatments	Skin	Nursing goals	General care	Sign off

Room:	Name:		Age/Sex:	Admit:
Code:	Allergies:		Isolation:	

Attending:	Consults:
Diagnosis:	PMH:

Na:	RBC:	Meds:
K:	WBC:	
Ca:	Hgb:	
Mg:	Hct:	
Ph:	Platelets:	
Cl:	INR:	
Glu:	PTT:	
CO2:	BUN:	
	Creat:	

Diagnostics:	IV:	Fluids:

Vitals:			Intake	Output
T:				
P:				
R:				
BP:				
O2:				

Neuro:	Neuro/CIWA	Cardio/Tele:	Pain Assess:	Pain Reassess:	Blood Sugar:
Resp:	Lungs/O2	DVT Prophylaxis:			
GI: Diet: Last BM: GU:		Skin:	Edema: Mobility:	Notes:	

| Assessment | Education | IV's/Lines | Care plan review | I&O's | Chart check |
| Reassessment | Treatments | Skin | Nursing goals | General care | Sign off |

Room:	Name:		Age/Sex:	Admit:

Code:	Allergies:		Isolation:

Attending:	Consults:

Diagnosis:	PMH:

Na:	RBC:	Meds:
K:	WBC:	
Ca:	Hgb:	
Mg:	Hct:	
Ph:	Platelets:	
Cl:	INR:	
Glu:	PTT:	
CO2:	BUN:	
	Creat:	

Diagnostics:	IV:	Fluids:

Vitals:			Intake	Output
T:				
P:				
R:				
BP:				
O2:				

Neuro:	Neuro/CIWA	Cardio/Tele:	Pain Assess:	Pain Reassess:	Blood Sugar:
Resp:	Lungs/O2	DVT Prophylaxis:			
GI: Diet: Last BM:		Skin:	Edema:	Notes:	
GU:			Mobility:		

| Assessment | Education | IV's/Lines | Care plan review | I&O's | Chart check |
| Reassessment | Treatments | Skin | Nursing goals | General care | Sign off |

Room:	Name:		Age/Sex:	Admit:

Code:	Allergies:		Isolation:

Attending:	Consults:

Diagnosis:	PMH:

Na:	RBC:	Meds:
K:	WBC:	
Ca:	Hgb:	
Mg:	Hct:	
Ph:	Platelets:	
Cl:	INR:	
Glu:	PTT:	
CO2:	BUN:	
	Creat:	

Diagnostics:	IV:	Fluids:

Vitals:			Intake	Output
T:				
P:				
R:				
BP:				
O2:				

Neuro:	Neuro/CIWA	Cardio/Tele:	Pain Assess:	Pain Reassess:	Blood Sugar:
Resp:	Lungs/O2				
		DVT Prophylaxis:			
GI: Diet: Last BM:		Skin:	Edema:	Notes:	
GU:			Mobility:		

Assessment	Education	IV's/Lines	Care plan review	I&O's	Chart check
Reassessment	Treatments	Skin	Nursing goals	General care	Sign off

Room:	Name:		Age/Sex:	Admit:
Code:	Allergies:		Isolation:	

Attending:	Consults:
Diagnosis:	PMH:

Na:	RBC:	Meds:
K:	WBC:	
Ca:	Hgb:	
Mg:	Hct:	
Ph:	Platelets:	
Cl:	INR:	
Glu:	PTT:	
CO2:	BUN:	
	Creat:	

Diagnostics:	IV:	Fluids:

Vitals:			Intake	Output
T:				
P:				
R:				
BP:				
O2:				

Neuro:	Neuro/CIWA	Cardio/Tele:	Pain Assess:	Pain Reassess:	Blood Sugar:
Resp:	Lungs/O2	DVT Prophylaxis:			
GI: Diet: Last BM:					
GU:		Skin:	Edema: Mobility:	Notes:	

Assessment	Education	IV's/Lines	Care plan review	I&O's	Chart check
Reassessment	Treatments	Skin	Nursing goals	General care	Sign off

Room:	Name:		Age/Sex:	Admit:

Code:	Allergies:		Isolation:

Attending:	Consults:

Diagnosis:	PMH:

Na:	RBC:	Meds:
K:	WBC:	
Ca:	Hgb:	
Mg:	Hct:	
Ph:	Platelets:	
Cl:	INR:	
Glu:	PTT:	
CO2:	BUN:	
	Creat:	

Diagnostics:	IV:	Fluids:

Vitals:			Intake	Output
T:				
P:				
R:				
BP:				
O2:				

Neuro:	Neuro/CIWA	Cardio/Tele:	Pain Assess:	Pain Reassess:	Blood Sugar:
Resp:	Lungs/O2	DVT Prophylaxis:			

GI:
  Diet:
  Last BM:
GU:
		Skin:	Edema:
			Mobility:
				Notes:	

Assessment	Education	IV's/Lines	Care plan review	I&O's	Chart check
Reassessment	Treatments	Skin	Nursing goals	General care	Sign off

Room:	Name:		Age/Sex:	Admit:
Code:	Allergies:			Isolation:

Attending:	Consults:

Diagnosis:	PMH:

Na:	RBC:	Meds:
K:	WBC:	
Ca:	Hgb:	
Mg:	Hct:	
Ph:	Platelets:	
Cl:	INR:	
Glu:	PTT:	
CO2:	BUN:	
	Creat:	

Diagnostics:	IV:	Fluids:

Vitals:			Intake	Output
T:				
P:				
R:				
BP:				
O2:				

Neuro:	Neuro/CIWA	Cardio/Tele:	Pain Assess:	Pain Reassess:	Blood Sugar:
Resp:	Lungs/O2	DVT Prophylaxis:			
GI: Diet: Last BM: GU:		Skin:	Edema: Mobility:	Notes:	

Assessment	Education	IV's/Lines	Care plan review	I&O's	Chart check
Reassessment	Treatments	Skin	Nursing goals	General care	Sign off

Room:	Name:		Age/Sex:	Admit:

Code:	Allergies:		Isolation:

Attending:	Consults:

Diagnosis:	PMH:

Na:	RBC:	Meds:
K:	WBC:	
Ca:	Hgb:	
Mg:	Hct:	
Ph:	Platelets:	
Cl:	INR:	
Glu:	PTT:	
CO2:	BUN:	
	Creat:	

Diagnostics:	IV:	Fluids:

Vitals:			Intake	Output
T:				
P:				
R:				
BP:				
O2:				

Neuro:	Neuro/CIWA	Cardio/Tele:	Pain Assess:	Pain Reassess:	Blood Sugar:
Resp:	Lungs/O2	DVT Prophylaxis:			
GI:					
Diet:					
Last BM:		Skin:	Edema:	Notes:	
GU:			Mobility:		

| Assessment | Education | IV's/Lines | Care plan review | I&O's | Chart check |
| Reassessment | Treatments | Skin | Nursing goals | General care | Sign off |

Room:	Name:		Age/Sex:	Admit:
Code:	Allergies:		Isolation:	

Attending:	Consults:
Diagnosis:	PMH:

Na:	RBC:	Meds:
K:	WBC:	
Ca:	Hgb:	
Mg:	Hct:	
Ph:	Platelets:	
Cl:	INR:	
Glu:	PTT:	
CO2:	BUN:	
	Creat:	

Diagnostics:	IV:	Fluids:

Vitals:			Intake	Output
T:				
P:				
R:				
BP:				
O2:				

Neuro:	Neuro/CIWA	Cardio/Tele:	Pain Assess:	Pain Reassess:	Blood Sugar:
Resp:	Lungs/O2	DVT Prophylaxis:			

GI:
    Diet:
    Last BM:					

		Skin:	Edema:	Notes:	
GU:			Mobility:		

Assessment	Education	IV's/Lines	Care plan review	I&O's	Chart check
Reassessment	Treatments	Skin	Nursing goals	General care	Sign off

Room:	Name:		Age/Sex:	Admit:
Code:	Allergies:			Isolation:

Attending:	Consults:
Diagnosis:	PMH:

Na:	RBC:	Meds:
K:	WBC:	
Ca:	Hgb:	
Mg:	Hct:	
Ph:	Platelets:	
Cl:	INR:	
Glu:	PTT:	
CO2:	BUN:	
	Creat:	

Diagnostics:	IV:	Fluids:

Vitals:			Intake	Output
T:				
P:				
R:				
BP:				
O2:				

Neuro:	Neuro/CIWA	Cardio/Tele:	Pain Assess:	Pain Reassess:	Blood Sugar:
Resp:	Lungs/O2	DVT Prophylaxis:			
GI: Diet: Last BM:		Skin:	Edema:	Notes:	
GU:			Mobility:		

Assessment	Education	IV's/Lines	Care plan review	I&O's	Chart check
Reassessment	Treatments	Skin	Nursing goals	General care	Sign off

Room:	Name:		Age/Sex:	Admit:
Code:	Allergies:			Isolation:

Attending:

Consults:

Diagnosis:

PMH:

Na:	RBC:	Meds:
K:	WBC:	
Ca:	Hgb:	
Mg:	Hct:	
Ph:	Platelets:	
Cl:	INR:	
Glu:	PTT:	
CO2:	BUN:	
	Creat:	

Diagnostics:	IV:	Fluids:

Vitals:			Intake	Output
T:				
P:				
R:				
BP:				
O2:				

Neuro:	Neuro/CIWA	Cardio/Tele:	Pain Assess:	Pain Reassess:	Blood Sugar:
Resp:	Lungs/O2	DVT Prophylaxis:			
GI: Diet: Last BM: GU:		Skin:	Edema: Mobility:	Notes:	

Assessment	Education	IV's/Lines	Care plan review	I&O's	Chart check
Reassessment	Treatments	Skin	Nursing goals	General care	Sign off

Room:	Name:		Age/Sex:	Admit:
Code:	Allergies:			Isolation:

Attending:	Consults:
Diagnosis:	PMH:

Na:	RBC:	Meds:
K:	WBC:	
Ca:	Hgb:	
Mg:	Hct:	
Ph:	Platelets:	
Cl:	INR:	
Glu:	PTT:	
CO2:	BUN:	
	Creat:	

Diagnostics:	IV:	Fluids:

Vitals:			Intake	Output
T:				
P:				
R:				
BP:				
O2:				

Neuro:	Neuro/CIWA	Cardio/Tele:	Pain Assess:	Pain Reassess:	Blood Sugar:
Resp:	Lungs/O2				
		DVT Prophylaxis:			
GI: Diet: Last BM:		Skin:	Edema:	Notes:	
GU:			Mobility:		

Assessment	Education	IV's/Lines	Care plan review	I&O's	Chart check
Reassessment	Treatments	Skin	Nursing goals	General care	Sign off

Room:	Name:		Age/Sex:	Admit:
Code:	Allergies:			Isolation:

Attending:	Consults:
Diagnosis:	PMH:

Na:	RBC:	Meds:
K:	WBC:	
Ca:	Hgb:	
Mg:	Hct:	
Ph:	Platelets:	
Cl:	INR:	
Glu:	PTT:	
CO2:	BUN:	
	Creat:	

Diagnostics:	IV:	Fluids:

Vitals:			Intake	Output
T:				
P:				
R:				
BP:				
O2:				

Neuro: Neuro/CIWA	Cardio/Tele:	Pain Assess:	Pain Reassess:	Blood Sugar:
Resp: Lungs/O2	DVT Prophylaxis:			
GI: Diet: Last BM: GU:	Skin:	Edema: Mobility:	Notes:	

Assessment	Education	IV's/Lines	Care plan review	I&O's	Chart check
Reassessment	Treatments	Skin	Nursing goals	General care	Sign off

Room:	Name:		Age/Sex:	Admit:

Code:	Allergies:		Isolation:

Attending:	Consults:

Diagnosis:	PMH:

Na:	RBC:	Meds:
K:	WBC:	
Ca:	Hgb:	
Mg:	Hct:	
Ph:	Platelets:	
Cl:	INR:	
Glu:	PTT:	
CO2:	BUN:	
	Creat:	

Diagnostics:	IV:	Fluids:

Vitals:			Intake	Output
T:				
P:				
R:				
BP:				
O2:				

Neuro:	Neuro/CIWA	Cardio/Tele:	Pain Assess:	Pain Reassess:	Blood Sugar:
Resp:	Lungs/O2	DVT Prophylaxis:			
GI: Diet: Last BM:					
GU:		Skin:	Edema: Mobility:	Notes:	

Assessment　　　Education　　　IV's/Lines　　　Care plan review　　　I&O's　　　Chart check
Reassessment　　Treatments　　　Skin　　　Nursing goals　　　General care　　　Sign off

Room:	Name:		Age/Sex:	Admit:
Code:	Allergies:			Isolation:

Attending:		Consults:
Diagnosis:		PMH:

Na:	RBC:	Meds:
K:	WBC:	
Ca:	Hgb:	
Mg:	Hct:	
Ph:	Platelets:	
Cl:	INR:	
Glu:	PTT:	
CO2:	BUN:	
	Creat:	

Diagnostics:	IV:	Fluids:

Vitals:			Intake	Output
T:				
P:				
R:				
BP:				
O2:				

Neuro:	Neuro/CIWA	Cardio/Tele:	Pain Assess:	Pain Reassess:	Blood Sugar:
Resp:	Lungs/O2	DVT Prophylaxis:			
GI: Diet: Last BM: GU:		Skin:	Edema: Mobility:	Notes:	

Assessment	Education	IV's/Lines	Care plan review	I&O's	Chart check
Reassessment	Treatments	Skin	Nursing goals	General care	Sign off

Room:	Name:		Age/Sex:	Admit:

Code:	Allergies:		Isolation:

Attending:

Consults:

Diagnosis:

PMH:

Na:	RBC:	Meds:
K:	WBC:	
Ca:	Hgb:	
Mg:	Hct:	
Ph:	Platelets:	
Cl:	INR:	
Glu:	PTT:	
CO2:	BUN:	
	Creat:	

Diagnostics:	IV:	Fluids:

Vitals:			Intake	Output
T:				
P:				
R:				
BP:				
O2:				

Neuro:	Neuro/CIWA	Cardio/Tele:	Pain Assess:	Pain Reassess:	Blood Sugar:
Resp:	Lungs/O2				
		DVT Prophylaxis:			
GI: Diet: Last BM:		Skin:	Edema:	Notes:	
GU:			Mobility:		

Assessment	Education	IV's/Lines	Care plan review	I&O's	Chart check
Reassessment	Treatments	Skin	Nursing goals	General care	Sign off

Room:	Name:		Age/Sex:	Admit:

Code:	Allergies:	Isolation:

Attending:	Consults:

Diagnosis:	PMH:

Na:	RBC:	Meds:
K:	WBC:	
Ca:	Hgb:	
Mg:	Hct:	
Ph:	Platelets:	
Cl:	INR:	
Glu:	PTT:	
CO2:	BUN:	
	Creat:	

Diagnostics:	IV:	Fluids:

Vitals:			Intake	Output
T:				
P:				
R:				
BP:				
O2:				

Neuro:	Neuro/CIWA	Cardio/Tele:	Pain Assess:	Pain Reassess:	Blood Sugar:
Resp:	Lungs/O2	DVT Prophylaxis:			
GI: Diet: Last BM: GU:		Skin:	Edema: Mobility:	Notes:	

Assessment	Education	IV's/Lines	Care plan review	I&O's	Chart check
Reassessment	Treatments	Skin	Nursing goals	General care	Sign off

Room:	Name:		Age/Sex:	Admit:

Code:	Allergies:		Isolation:

Attending:	Consults:

Diagnosis:	PMH:

Na:	RBC:	Meds:
K:	WBC:	
Ca:	Hgb:	
Mg:	Hct:	
Ph:	Platelets:	
Cl:	INR:	
Glu:	PTT:	
CO2:	BUN:	
	Creat:	

Diagnostics:	IV:	Fluids:

Vitals:			Intake	Output
T:				
P:				
R:				
BP:				
O2:				

Neuro:	Neuro/CIWA	Cardio/Tele:	Pain Assess:	Pain Reassess:	Blood Sugar:
Resp:	Lungs/O2				
		DVT Prophylaxis:			
GI:					
Diet:					
Last BM:		Skin:	Edema:	Notes:	
GU:			Mobility:		

| Assessment | Education | IV's/Lines | Care plan review | I&O's | Chart check |
| Reassessment | Treatments | Skin | Nursing goals | General care | Sign off |

Room:	Name:		Age/Sex:	Admit:

Code:	Allergies:		Isolation:

Attending:	Consults:

Diagnosis:	PMH:

Na:	RBC:	Meds:
K:	WBC:	
Ca:	Hgb:	
Mg:	Hct:	
Ph:	Platelets:	
Cl:	INR:	
Glu:	PTT:	
CO2:	BUN:	
	Creat:	

Diagnostics:	IV:	Fluids:

Vitals:			Intake	Output
T:				
P:				
R:				
BP:				
O2:				

Neuro:	Neuro/CIWA	Cardio/Tele:	Pain Assess:	Pain Reassess:	Blood Sugar:
Resp:	Lungs/O2	DVT Prophylaxis:			
GI: Diet: Last BM: GU:		Skin:	Edema: Mobility:	Notes:	

Assessment   Education   IV's/Lines   Care plan review   I&O's   Chart check
Reassessment   Treatments   Skin   Nursing goals   General care   Sign off

Room:	Name:		Age/Sex:	Admit:

Code:	Allergies:	Isolation:

Attending:	Consults:

Diagnosis:	PMH:

Na:	RBC:	Meds:
K:	WBC:	
Ca:	Hgb:	
Mg:	Hct:	
Ph:	Platelets:	
Cl:	INR:	
Glu:	PTT:	
CO2:	BUN:	
	Creat:	

Diagnostics:	IV:	Fluids:

Vitals:			Intake	Output
T:				
P:				
R:				
BP:				
O2:				

Neuro:	Neuro/CIWA	Cardio/Tele:	Pain Assess:	Pain Reassess:	Blood Sugar:
Resp:	Lungs/O2	DVT Prophylaxis:			
GI: Diet: Last BM:		Skin:	Edema:	Notes:	
GU:			Mobility:		

Assessment	Education	IV's/Lines	Care plan review	I&O's	Chart check
Reassessment	Treatments	Skin	Nursing goals	General care	Sign off

Room:	Name:		Age/Sex:	Admit:
Code:	Allergies:		Isolation:	

Attending:	Consults:
Diagnosis:	PMH:

Na:	RBC:	Meds:
K:	WBC:	
Ca:	Hgb:	
Mg:	Hct:	
Ph:	Platelets:	
Cl:	INR:	
Glu:	PTT:	
CO2:	BUN:	
	Creat:	

Diagnostics:	IV:	Fluids:

Vitals:			Intake	Output
T:				
P:				
R:				
BP:				
O2:				

Neuro:	Neuro/CIWA	Cardio/Tele:	Pain Assess:	Pain Reassess:	Blood Sugar:
Resp:	Lungs/O2	DVT Prophylaxis:			
GI: Diet: Last BM: GU:		Skin:	Edema: Mobility:	Notes:	

Assessment	Education	IV's/Lines	Care plan review	I&O's	Chart check
Reassessment	Treatments	Skin	Nursing goals	General care	Sign off

Room:	Name:		Age/Sex:	Admit:

Code:	Allergies:	Isolation:

Attending:	Consults:

Diagnosis:	PMH:

Na:	RBC:	Meds:
K:	WBC:	
Ca:	Hgb:	
Mg:	Hct:	
Ph:	Platelets:	
Cl:	INR:	
Glu:	PTT:	
CO2:	BUN:	
	Creat:	

Diagnostics:	IV:	Fluids:

Vitals:			Intake	Output
T:				
P:				
R:				
BP:				
O2:				

Neuro:	Neuro/CIWA	Cardio/Tele:	Pain Assess:	Pain Reassess:	Blood Sugar:
Resp:	Lungs/O2	DVT Prophylaxis:			
GI: Diet: Last BM: GU:		Skin:	Edema: Mobility:	Notes:	

Assessment Reassessment	Education Treatments	IV's/Lines Skin	Care plan review Nursing goals	I&O's General care	Chart check Sign off

Room:	Name:		Age/Sex:	Admit:
Code:	Allergies:			Isolation:

Attending:	Consults:

Diagnosis:	PMH:

Na:	RBC:	Meds:
K:	WBC:	
Ca:	Hgb:	
Mg:	Hct:	
Ph:	Platelets:	
Cl:	INR:	
Glu:	PTT:	
CO2:	BUN:	
	Creat:	

Diagnostics:	IV:	Fluids:

Vitals:			Intake	Output
T:				
P:				
R:				
BP:				
O2:				

Neuro:	Neuro/CIWA	Cardio/Tele:	Pain Assess:	Pain Reassess:	Blood Sugar:
Resp:	Lungs/O2	DVT Prophylaxis:			
GI: Diet: Last BM:		Skin:	Edema:	Notes:	
GU:			Mobility:		

Assessment   Education   IV's/Lines   Care plan review   I&O's   Chart check
Reassessment   Treatments   Skin   Nursing goals   General care   Sign off

Room:	Name:		Age/Sex:	Admit:

Code:	Allergies:	Isolation:

Attending:	Consults:

Diagnosis:	PMH:

Na:	RBC:	Meds:
K:	WBC:	
Ca:	Hgb:	
Mg:	Hct:	
Ph:	Platelets:	
Cl:	INR:	
Glu:	PTT:	
CO2:	BUN:	
	Creat:	

Diagnostics:	IV:	Fluids:

Vitals:			Intake	Output
T:				
P:				
R:				
BP:				
O2:				

Neuro:	Neuro/CIWA	Cardio/Tele:	Pain Assess:	Pain Reassess:	Blood Sugar:
Resp:	Lungs/O2				
		DVT Prophylaxis:			
GI: Diet: Last BM:		Skin:	Edema:	Notes:	
GU:			Mobility:		

Assessment Reassessment	Education Treatments	IV's/Lines Skin	Care plan review Nursing goals	I&O's General care	Chart check Sign off

Room:	Name:		Age/Sex:	Admit:
Code:	Allergies:		Isolation:	

Attending:	Consults:
Diagnosis:	PMH:

Na:	RBC:	Meds:
K:	WBC:	
Ca:	Hgb:	
Mg:	Hct:	
Ph:	Platelets:	
Cl:	INR:	
Glu:	PTT:	
CO2:	BUN:	
	Creat:	

Diagnostics:	IV:	Fluids:

Vitals:			Intake	Output
T:				
P:				
R:				
BP:				
O2:				

Neuro:	Neuro/CIWA	Cardio/Tele:	Pain Assess:	Pain Reassess:	Blood Sugar:
Resp:	Lungs/O2	DVT Prophylaxis:			
GI: Diet: Last BM:		Skin:	Edema:	Notes:	
GU:			Mobility:		

Assessment	Education	IV's/Lines	Care plan review	I&O's	Chart check
Reassessment	Treatments	Skin	Nursing goals	General care	Sign off

Room:	Name:		Age/Sex:	Admit:
Code:	Allergies:			Isolation:

Attending:	Consults:
Diagnosis:	PMH:

Na:	RBC:	Meds:
K:	WBC:	
Ca:	Hgb:	
Mg:	Hct:	
Ph:	Platelets:	
Cl:	INR:	
Glu:	PTT:	
CO2:	BUN:	
	Creat:	

Diagnostics:	IV:	Fluids:

Vitals:			Intake	Output
T:				
P:				
R:				
BP:				
O2:				

Neuro:	Neuro/CIWA	Cardio/Tele:	Pain Assess:	Pain Reassess:	Blood Sugar:
Resp:	Lungs/O2	DVT Prophylaxis:			
GI: Diet: Last BM: GU:		Skin:	Edema: Mobility:	Notes:	

Assessment	Education	IV's/Lines	Care plan review	I&O's	Chart check
Reassessment	Treatments	Skin	Nursing goals	General care	Sign off

Room:	Name:		Age/Sex:	Admit:
Code:	Allergies:			Isolation:

Attending:	Consults:
Diagnosis:	PMH:

Na:	RBC:	Meds:
K:	WBC:	
Ca:	Hgb:	
Mg:	Hct:	
Ph:	Platelets:	
Cl:	INR:	
Glu:	PTT:	
CO2:	BUN:	
	Creat:	

Diagnostics:		IV:	Fluids:

Vitals:			Intake	Output
T:				
P:				
R:				
BP:				
O2:				

Neuro:	Neuro/CIWA	Cardio/Tele:	Pain Assess:	Pain Reassess:	Blood Sugar:
Resp:	Lungs/O2	DVT Prophylaxis:			
GI: Diet: Last BM: GU:		Skin:	Edema: Mobility:	Notes:	

Assessment	Education	IV's/Lines	Care plan review	I&O's	Chart check
Reassessment	Treatments	Skin	Nursing goals	General care	Sign off

Room:	Name:		Age/Sex:	Admit:

Code:	Allergies:		Isolation:

Attending:	Consults:

Diagnosis:	PMH:

Na:	RBC:	Meds:
K:	WBC:	
Ca:	Hgb:	
Mg:	Hct:	
Ph:	Platelets:	
Cl:	INR:	
Glu:	PTT:	
CO2:	BUN:	
	Creat:	

Diagnostics:	IV:	Fluids:

Vitals:			Intake	Output
T:				
P:				
R:				
BP:				
O2:				

Neuro:	Neuro/CIWA	Cardio/Tele:	Pain Assess:	Pain Reassess:	Blood Sugar:
Resp:	Lungs/O2	DVT Prophylaxis:			
GI: Diet: Last BM: GU:		Skin:	Edema: Mobility:	Notes:	

Assessment	Education	IV's/Lines	Care plan review	I&O's	Chart check
Reassessment	Treatments	Skin	Nursing goals	General care	Sign off

Room:	Name:		Age/Sex:	Admit:
Code:	Allergies:			Isolation:

Attending:	Consults:

Diagnosis:	PMH:

Na:	RBC:	Meds:
K:	WBC:	
Ca:	Hgb:	
Mg:	Hct:	
Ph:	Platelets:	
Cl:	INR:	
Glu:	PTT:	
CO2:	BUN:	
	Creat:	

Diagnostics:	IV:	Fluids:

Vitals:			Intake	Output
T:				
P:				
R:				
BP:				
O2:				

Neuro:	Neuro/CIWA	Cardio/Tele:	Pain Assess:	Pain Reassess:	Blood Sugar:
Resp:	Lungs/O2				
		DVT Prophylaxis:			
GI: Diet: Last BM:		Skin:	Edema:	Notes:	
GU:			Mobility:		

Assessment	Education	IV's/Lines	Care plan review	I&O's	Chart check
Reassessment	Treatments	Skin	Nursing goals	General care	Sign off

Room:	Name:			Age/Sex:	Admit:
Code:	Allergies:				Isolation:

Attending:	Consults:
Diagnosis:	PMH:

Na:	RBC:	Meds:
K:	WBC:	
Ca:	Hgb:	
Mg:	Hct:	
Ph:	Platelets:	
Cl:	INR:	
Glu:	PTT:	
CO2:	BUN:	
	Creat:	

Diagnostics:	IV:	Fluids:

Vitals:			Intake	Output
T:				
P:				
R:				
BP:				
O2:				

Neuro:	Neuro/CIWA	Cardio/Tele:	Pain Assess:	Pain Reassess:	Blood Sugar:
Resp:	Lungs/O2	DVT Prophylaxis:			
GI: Diet: Last BM:					
GU:		Skin:	Edema:	Notes:	
			Mobility:		

Assessment Education IV's/Lines Care plan review I&O's Chart check
Reassessment Treatments Skin Nursing goals General care Sign off

Room:	Name:		Age/Sex:	Admit:
Code:	Allergies:			Isolation:

Attending:	Consults:
Diagnosis:	PMH:

Na:	RBC:	Meds:
K:	WBC:	
Ca:	Hgb:	
Mg:	Hct:	
Ph:	Platelets:	
Cl:	INR:	
Glu:	PTT:	
CO2:	BUN:	
	Creat:	

Diagnostics:	IV:	Fluids:

Vitals:			Intake	Output
T:				
P:				
R:				
BP:				
O2:				

Neuro:	Neuro/CIWA	Cardio/Tele:	Pain Assess:	Pain Reassess:	Blood Sugar:
Resp:	Lungs/O2	DVT Prophylaxis:			
GI: Diet: Last BM: GU:		Skin:	Edema: Mobility:	Notes:	

Assessment   Education   IV's/Lines   Care plan review   I&O's   Chart check
Reassessment   Treatments   Skin   Nursing goals   General care   Sign off

Room:	Name:		Age/Sex:	Admit:

Code:	Allergies:	Isolation:

Attending:	Consults:

Diagnosis:	PMH:

Na:	RBC:	Meds:
K:	WBC:	
Ca:	Hgb:	
Mg:	Hct:	
Ph:	Platelets:	
Cl:	INR:	
Glu:	PTT:	
CO2:	BUN:	
	Creat:	

Diagnostics:	IV:	Fluids:

Vitals:			Intake	Output
T:				
P:				
R:				
BP:				
O2:				

Neuro:	Neuro/CIWA	Cardio/Tele:	Pain Assess:	Pain Reassess:	Blood Sugar:
Resp:	Lungs/O2				
		DVT Prophylaxis:			
GI:		Skin:	Edema:	Notes:	
Diet:					
Last BM:			Mobility:		
GU:					

Assessment	Education	IV's/Lines	Care plan review	I&O's	Chart check
Reassessment	Treatments	Skin	Nursing goals	General care	Sign off

Room:	Name:		Age/Sex:	Admit:
Code:	Allergies:		Isolation:	

Attending:	Consults:
Diagnosis:	PMH:

Na:	RBC:	Meds:
K:	WBC:	
Ca:	Hgb:	
Mg:	Hct:	
Ph:	Platelets:	
Cl:	INR:	
Glu:	PTT:	
CO2:	BUN:	
	Creat:	

Diagnostics:	IV:	Fluids:

Vitals:			Intake	Output
T:				
P:				
R:				
BP:				
O2:				

Neuro:	Neuro/CIWA	Cardio/Tele:	Pain Assess:	Pain Reassess:	Blood Sugar:
Resp:	Lungs/O2	DVT Prophylaxis:			
GI: Diet: Last BM:		Skin:	Edema:	Notes:	
GU:			Mobility:		

Assessment	Education	IV's/Lines	Care plan review	I&O's	Chart check
Reassessment	Treatments	Skin	Nursing goals	General care	Sign off

Room:	Name:			Age/Sex:	Admit:
Code:	Allergies:				Isolation:

Attending:	Consults:
Diagnosis:	PMH:

Na:	RBC:	Meds:
K:	WBC:	
Ca:	Hgb:	
Mg:	Hct:	
Ph:	Platelets:	
Cl:	INR:	
Glu:	PTT:	
CO2:	BUN:	
	Creat:	

Diagnostics:	IV:	Fluids:

Vitals:			Intake	Output
T:				
P:				
R:				
BP:				
O2:				

Neuro:	Neuro/CIWA	Cardio/Tele:	Pain Assess:	Pain Reassess:	Blood Sugar:
Resp:	Lungs/O2	DVT Prophylaxis:			
GI: Diet: Last BM: GU:		Skin:	Edema: Mobility:	Notes:	

| Assessment | Education | IV's/Lines | Care plan review | I&O's | Chart check |
| Reassessment | Treatments | Skin | Nursing goals | General care | Sign off |

Room:	Name:		Age/Sex:	Admit:
Code:	Allergies:			Isolation:

Attending:	Consults:

Diagnosis:	PMH:

Na:	RBC:	Meds:
K:	WBC:	
Ca:	Hgb:	
Mg:	Hct:	
Ph:	Platelets:	
Cl:	INR:	
Glu:	PTT:	
CO2:	BUN:	
	Creat:	

Diagnostics:	IV:	Fluids:

Vitals:			Intake	Output
T:				
P:				
R:				
BP:				
O2:				

Neuro: Neuro/CIWA	Cardio/Tele:	Pain Assess:	Pain Reassess:	Blood Sugar:
Resp: Lungs/O2	DVT Prophylaxis:			
GI: Diet: Last BM:	Skin:	Edema:	Notes:	
GU:		Mobility:		

Assessment   Education   IV's/Lines   Care plan review   I&O's   Chart check
Reassessment   Treatments   Skin   Nursing goals   General care   Sign off

Room:	Name:		Age/Sex:	Admit:

Code:	Allergies:		Isolation:

Attending:	Consults:

Diagnosis:	PMH:

Na:	RBC:	Meds:
K:	WBC:	
Ca:	Hgb:	
Mg:	Hct:	
Ph:	Platelets:	
Cl:	INR:	
Glu:	PTT:	
CO2:	BUN:	
	Creat:	

Diagnostics:	IV:	Fluids:

Vitals:			Intake	Output
T:				
P:				
R:				
BP:				
O2:				

Neuro:	Neuro/CIWA	Cardio/Tele:	Pain Assess:	Pain Reassess:	Blood Sugar:
Resp:	Lungs/O2	DVT Prophylaxis:			
GI: Diet: Last BM:		Skin:	Edema:	Notes:	
GU:			Mobility:		

Assessment　　　　Education　　　　IV's/Lines　　　　Care plan review　　　　I&O's　　　　Chart check
Reassessment　　　Treatments　　　　Skin　　　　　　Nursing goals　　　　General care　　　Sign off

Room:	Name:		Age/Sex:	Admit:
Code:	Allergies:		Isolation:	

Attending:	Consults:
Diagnosis:	PMH:

Na:	RBC:	Meds:
K:	WBC:	
Ca:	Hgb:	
Mg:	Hct:	
Ph:	Platelets:	
Cl:	INR:	
Glu:	PTT:	
CO2:	BUN:	
	Creat:	

Diagnostics:	IV:	Fluids:

Vitals:			Intake	Output
T:				
P:				
R:				
BP:				
O2:				

Neuro:	Neuro/CIWA	Cardio/Tele:	Pain Assess:	Pain Reassess:	Blood Sugar:
Resp:	Lungs/O2	DVT Prophylaxis:			
GI:					
Diet:					
Last BM:		Skin:	Edema:	Notes:	
GU:			Mobility:		

Assessment	Education	IV's/Lines	Care plan review	I&O's	Chart check
Reassessment	Treatments	Skin	Nursing goals	General care	Sign off

Room:	Name:		Age/Sex:	Admit:

Code:	Allergies:	Isolation:

Attending:	Consults:

Diagnosis:	PMH:

Na:	RBC:	Meds:
K:	WBC:	
Ca:	Hgb:	
Mg:	Hct:	
Ph:	Platelets:	
Cl:	INR:	
Glu:	PTT:	
CO2:	BUN:	
	Creat:	

Diagnostics:	IV:	Fluids:

Vitals:			Intake	Output
T:				
P:				
R:				
BP:				
O2:				

Neuro:	Neuro/CIWA	Cardio/Tele:	Pain Assess:	Pain Reassess:	Blood Sugar:
Resp:	Lungs/O2				
		DVT Prophylaxis:			

GI:
  Diet:
  Last BM:
GU:
		Skin:	Edema:
			Mobility:
				Notes:	

Assessment	Education	IV's/Lines	Care plan review	I&O's	Chart check
Reassessment	Treatments	Skin	Nursing goals	General care	Sign off

Room:	Name:		Age/Sex:	Admit:

Code:	Allergies:		Isolation:

Attending:	Consults:

Diagnosis:	PMH:

Na:	RBC:	Meds:
K:	WBC:	
Ca:	Hgb:	
Mg:	Hct:	
Ph:	Platelets:	
Cl:	INR:	
Glu:	PTT:	
CO2:	BUN:	
	Creat:	

Diagnostics:	IV:	Fluids:

Vitals:			Intake	Output
T:				
P:				
R:				
BP:				
O2:				

Neuro:	Neuro/CIWA	Cardio/Tele:	Pain Assess:	Pain Reassess:	Blood Sugar:
Resp:	Lungs/O2	DVT Prophylaxis:			
GI: 　Diet: 　Last BM: GU:		Skin:	Edema: Mobility:	Notes:	

Assessment	Education	IV's/Lines	Care plan review	I&O's	Chart check
Reassessment	Treatments	Skin	Nursing goals	General care	Sign off

Room:	Name:		Age/Sex:	Admit:
Code:	Allergies:			Isolation:

Attending:	Consults:
Diagnosis:	PMH:

Na:	RBC:	Meds:
K:	WBC:	
Ca:	Hgb:	
Mg:	Hct:	
Ph:	Platelets:	
Cl:	INR:	
Glu:	PTT:	
CO2:	BUN:	
	Creat:	

Diagnostics:	IV:	Fluids:

Vitals:			Intake	Output
T:				
P:				
R:				
BP:				
O2:				

Neuro:	Neuro/CIWA	Cardio/Tele:	Pain Assess:	Pain Reassess:	Blood Sugar:
Resp:	Lungs/O2				
		DVT Prophylaxis:			
GI: Diet: Last BM:		Skin:	Edema:	Notes:	
GU:			Mobility:		

Assessment	Education	IV's/Lines	Care plan review	I&O's	Chart check
Reassessment	Treatments	Skin	Nursing goals	General care	Sign off

Room:	Name:		Age/Sex:	Admit:
Code:	Allergies:		Isolation:	

Attending:	Consults:
Diagnosis:	PMH:

Na:	RBC:	Meds:
K:	WBC:	
Ca:	Hgb:	
Mg:	Hct:	
Ph:	Platelets:	
Cl:	INR:	
Glu:	PTT:	
CO2:	BUN:	
	Creat:	

Diagnostics:	IV:	Fluids:

Vitals:			Intake	Output
T:				
P:				
R:				
BP:				
O2:				

Neuro:	Neuro/CIWA	Cardio/Tele:	Pain Assess:	Pain Reassess:	Blood Sugar:
Resp:	Lungs/O2				
GI: Diet: Last BM:		DVT Prophylaxis:			
GU:		Skin:	Edema:	Notes:	
			Mobility:		

Assessment	Education	IV's/Lines	Care plan review	I&O's	Chart check
Reassessment	Treatments	Skin	Nursing goals	General care	Sign off

Room:	Name:		Age/Sex:	Admit:
Code:	Allergies:			Isolation:

Attending:	Consults:
Diagnosis:	PMH:

Na:	RBC:	Meds:
K:	WBC:	
Ca:	Hgb:	
Mg:	Hct:	
Ph:	Platelets:	
Cl:	INR:	
Glu:	PTT:	
CO2:	BUN:	
	Creat:	

Diagnostics:	IV:	Fluids:

Vitals:			Intake	Output
T:				
P:				
R:				
BP:				
O2:				

Neuro:	Neuro/CIWA	Cardio/Tele:	Pain Assess:	Pain Reassess:	Blood Sugar:
Resp:	Lungs/O2	DVT Prophylaxis:			
GI: Diet: Last BM:		Skin:	Edema:	Notes:	
GU:			Mobility:		

Assessment   Education   IV's/Lines   Care plan review   I&O's   Chart check
Reassessment   Treatments   Skin   Nursing goals   General care   Sign off

Room:	Name:		Age/Sex:	Admit:

Code:	Allergies:	Isolation:

Attending:	Consults:

Diagnosis:	PMH:

Na:	RBC:	Meds:
K:	WBC:	
Ca:	Hgb:	
Mg:	Hct:	
Ph:	Platelets:	
Cl:	INR:	
Glu:	PTT:	
CO2:	BUN:	
	Creat:	

Diagnostics:	IV:	Fluids:

Vitals:			Intake	Output
T:				
P:				
R:				
BP:				
O2:				

Neuro:	Neuro/CIWA	Cardio/Tele:	Pain Assess:	Pain Reassess:	Blood Sugar:
Resp:	Lungs/O2	DVT Prophylaxis:			
GI: Diet: Last BM:					
GU:		Skin:	Edema: Mobility:	Notes:	

Assessment	Education	IV's/Lines	Care plan review	I&O's	Chart check
Reassessment	Treatments	Skin	Nursing goals	General care	Sign off

Room:	Name:		Age/Sex:	Admit:

Code:	Allergies:		Isolation:

Attending:	Consults:

Diagnosis:	PMH:

Na:	RBC:	Meds:
K:	WBC:	
Ca:	Hgb:	
Mg:	Hct:	
Ph:	Platelets:	
Cl:	INR:	
Glu:	PTT:	
CO2:	BUN:	
	Creat:	

Diagnostics:	IV:	Fluids:

Vitals:			Intake	Output
T:				
P:				
R:				
BP:				
O2:				

Neuro:	Neuro/CIWA	Cardio/Tele:	Pain Assess:	Pain Reassess:	Blood Sugar:
Resp:	Lungs/O2	DVT Prophylaxis:			

GI:
  Diet:
  Last BM:
GU:
		Skin:	Edema:
			Mobility:
				Notes:	

Assessment	Education	IV's/Lines	Care plan review	I&O's	Chart check
Reassessment	Treatments	Skin	Nursing goals	General care	Sign off

Room:	Name:		Age/Sex:	Admit:
Code:	Allergies:		Isolation:	

Attending:	Consults:
Diagnosis:	PMH:

Na:	RBC:	Meds:
K:	WBC:	
Ca:	Hgb:	
Mg:	Hct:	
Ph:	Platelets:	
Cl:	INR:	
Glu:	PTT:	
CO2:	BUN:	
	Creat:	

Diagnostics:	IV:	Fluids:

Vitals:			Intake	Output
T:				
P:				
R:				
BP:				
O2:				

Neuro:	Neuro/CIWA	Cardio/Tele:	Pain Assess:	Pain Reassess:	Blood Sugar:
Resp:	Lungs/O2	DVT Prophylaxis:			
GI: Diet: Last BM:		Skin:	Edema:	Notes:	
GU:			Mobility:		

Assessment	Education	IV's/Lines	Care plan review	I&O's	Chart check
Reassessment	Treatments	Skin	Nursing goals	General care	Sign off

Room:	Name:		Age/Sex:	Admit:
Code:	Allergies:			Isolation:

Attending:	Consults:

Diagnosis:	PMH:

Na:	RBC:	Meds:
K:	WBC:	
Ca:	Hgb:	
Mg:	Hct:	
Ph:	Platelets:	
Cl:	INR:	
Glu:	PTT:	
CO_2:	BUN:	
	Creat:	

Diagnostics:	IV:	Fluids:

Vitals:			Intake	Output
T:				
P:				
R:				
BP:				
O2:				

Neuro:	Neuro/CIWA	Cardio/Tele:	Pain Assess:	Pain Reassess:	Blood Sugar:
Resp:	Lungs/O2	DVT Prophylaxis:			

GI:
  Diet:
  Last BM:
GU:
		Skin:	Edema:	Notes:	

			Mobility:		

Assessment	Education	IV's/Lines	Care plan review	I&O's	Chart check
Reassessment	Treatments	Skin	Nursing goals	General care	Sign off

Room:	Name:		Age/Sex:	Admit:

Code:	Allergies:		Isolation:

Attending:	Consults:

Diagnosis:	PMH:

Na:	RBC:	Meds:
K:	WBC:	
Ca:	Hgb:	
Mg:	Hct:	
Ph:	Platelets:	
Cl:	INR:	
Glu:	PTT:	
CO2:	BUN:	
	Creat:	

Diagnostics:	IV:	Fluids:

Vitals:			Intake	Output
T:				
P:				
R:				
BP:				
O2:				

Neuro:	Neuro/CIWA	Cardio/Tele:	Pain Assess:	Pain Reassess:	Blood Sugar:
Resp:	Lungs/O2	DVT Prophylaxis:			
GI: Diet: Last BM: GU:		Skin:	Edema: Mobility:	Notes:	

Assessment   Education   IV's/Lines   Care plan review   I&O's   Chart check
Reassessment   Treatments   Skin   Nursing goals   General care   Sign off

Room:	Name:			Age/Sex:	Admit:

Code:	Allergies:		Isolation:

Attending:	Consults:

Diagnosis:	PMH:

Na:	RBC:	Meds:
K:	WBC:	
Ca:	Hgb:	
Mg:	Hct:	
Ph:	Platelets:	
Cl:	INR:	
Glu:	PTT:	
CO2:	BUN:	
	Creat:	

Diagnostics:	IV:	Fluids:

Vitals:			Intake	Output
T:				
P:				
R:				
BP:				
O2:				

Neuro:	Neuro/CIWA	Cardio/Tele:	Pain Assess:	Pain Reassess:	Blood Sugar:
Resp:	Lungs/O2				
		DVT Prophylaxis:			
GI:					
Diet:					
Last BM:		Skin:	Edema:	Notes:	
GU:			Mobility:		

Assessment   Education   IV's/Lines   Care plan review   I&O's   Chart check
Reassessment   Treatments   Skin   Nursing goals   General care   Sign off

Room:	Name:		Age/Sex:	Admit:

Code:	Allergies:		Isolation:

Attending:	Consults:

Diagnosis:	PMH:

Na:	RBC:	Meds:
K:	WBC:	
Ca:	Hgb:	
Mg:	Hct:	
Ph:	Platelets:	
Cl:	INR:	
Glu:	PTT:	
CO2:	BUN:	
	Creat:	

Diagnostics:	IV:	Fluids:

Vitals:			Intake	Output
T:				
P:				
R:				
BP:				
O2:				

Neuro:	Neuro/CIWA	Cardio/Tele:	Pain Assess:	Pain Reassess:	Blood Sugar:
Resp:	Lungs/O2	DVT Prophylaxis:			
GI: Diet: Last BM:		Skin:	Edema: Mobility:	Notes:	
GU:					

Assessment	Education	IV's/Lines	Care plan review	I&O's	Chart check
Reassessment	Treatments	Skin	Nursing goals	General care	Sign off

Room:	Name:		Age/Sex:	Admit:
Code:	Allergies:			Isolation:

Attending:	Consults:
Diagnosis:	PMH:

Na:	RBC:	Meds:
K:	WBC:	
Ca:	Hgb:	
Mg:	Hct:	
Ph:	Platelets:	
Cl:	INR:	
Glu:	PTT:	
CO2:	BUN:	
	Creat:	

Diagnostics:	IV:	Fluids:

Vitals:			Intake	Output
T:				
P:				
R:				
BP:				
O2:				

Neuro:	Neuro/CIWA	Cardio/Tele:	Pain Assess:	Pain Reassess:	Blood Sugar:
Resp:	Lungs/O2	DVT Prophylaxis:			
GI: Diet: Last BM: GU:		Skin:	Edema: Mobility:	Notes:	

Assessment   Education   IV's/Lines   Care plan review   I&O's   Chart check
Reassessment   Treatments   Skin   Nursing goals   General care   Sign off

Room:	Name:		Age/Sex:	Admit:

Code:	Allergies:		Isolation:

Attending:	Consults:

Diagnosis:	PMH:

Na:	RBC:	Meds:
K:	WBC:	
Ca:	Hgb:	
Mg:	Hct:	
Ph:	Platelets:	
Cl:	INR:	
Glu:	PTT:	
CO2:	BUN:	
	Creat:	

Diagnostics:	IV:	Fluids:

Vitals:			Intake	Output
T:				
P:				
R:				
BP:				
O2:				

Neuro:	Neuro/CIWA	Cardio/Tele:	Pain Assess:	Pain Reassess:	Blood Sugar:
Resp:	Lungs/O2	DVT Prophylaxis:			
GI: Diet: Last BM:		Skin:	Edema:	Notes:	
GU:			Mobility:		

Assessment　　　　Education　　　　IV's/Lines　　　　Care plan review　　　　I&O's　　　　Chart check
Reassessment　　　　Treatments　　　　Skin　　　　Nursing goals　　　　General care　　　　Sign off

Room:	Name:		Age/Sex:	Admit:
Code:	Allergies:			Isolation:

Attending:	Consults:
Diagnosis:	PMH:

Na:	RBC:	Meds:
K:	WBC:	
Ca:	Hgb:	
Mg:	Hct:	
Ph:	Platelets:	
Cl:	INR:	
Glu:	PTT:	
CO2:	BUN:	
	Creat:	

Diagnostics:	IV:	Fluids:

Vitals:			Intake	Output
T:				
P:				
R:				
BP:				
O2:				

Neuro:	Neuro/CIWA	Cardio/Tele:	Pain Assess:	Pain Reassess:	Blood Sugar:
Resp:	Lungs/O2	DVT Prophylaxis:			
GI: Diet: Last BM:					
GU:		Skin:	Edema:	Notes:	
			Mobility:		

Assessment	Education	IV's/Lines	Care plan review	I&O's	Chart check
Reassessment	Treatments	Skin	Nursing goals	General care	Sign off

Room:	Name:		Age/Sex:	Admit:
Code:	Allergies:		Isolation:	

Attending:	Consults:
Diagnosis:	PMH:

Na:	RBC:	Meds:
K:	WBC:	
Ca:	Hgb:	
Mg:	Hct:	
Ph:	Platelets:	
Cl:	INR:	
Glu:	PTT:	
CO2:	BUN:	
	Creat:	

Diagnostics:	IV:	Fluids:

Vitals:			Intake	Output
T:				
P:				
R:				
BP:				
O2:				

Neuro:	Neuro/CIWA	Cardio/Tele:	Pain Assess:	Pain Reassess:	Blood Sugar:
Resp:	Lungs/O2	DVT Prophylaxis:			
GI: Diet: Last BM:		Skin:	Edema:	Notes:	
GU:			Mobility:		

Assessment   Education   IV's/Lines   Care plan review   I&O's   Chart check
Reassessment   Treatments   Skin   Nursing goals   General care   Sign off

Room:	Name:		Age/Sex:	Admit:

Code:	Allergies:	Isolation:

Attending:

Consults:

Diagnosis:

PMH:

Na:	RBC:	Meds:
K:	WBC:	
Ca:	Hgb:	
Mg:	Hct:	
Ph:	Platelets:	
Cl:	INR:	
Glu:	PTT:	
CO2:	BUN:	
	Creat:	

Diagnostics:	IV:	Fluids:

Vitals:			Intake	Output
T:				
P:				
R:				
BP:				
O2:				

Neuro:	Neuro/CIWA	Cardio/Tele:	Pain Assess:	Pain Reassess:	Blood Sugar:
Resp:	Lungs/O2	DVT Prophylaxis:			
GI: Diet: Last BM: GU:		Skin:	Edema: Mobility:	Notes:	

Assessment   Education   IV's/Lines   Care plan review   I&O's   Chart check

Reassessment   Treatments   Skin   Nursing goals   General care   Sign off

Room:	Name:		Age/Sex:	Admit:

Code:	Allergies:		Isolation:

Attending:	Consults:

Diagnosis:	PMH:

Na:	RBC:	Meds:
K:	WBC:	
Ca:	Hgb:	
Mg:	Hct	
Ph:	Platelets:	
Cl:	INR:	
Glu:	PTT:	
CO2:	BUN:	
	Creat:	

Diagnostics:	IV:	Fluids:

Vitals:			Intake	Output
T:				
P:				
R:				
BP:				
O2:				

Neuro:	Neuro/CIWA	Cardio/Tele:	Pain Assess:	Pain Reassess:	Blood Sugar:
Resp:	Lungs/O2	DVT Prophylaxis:			

GI:
  Diet:
  Last BM:
GU:
		Skin:	Edema:
			Mobility:
				Notes:	

Assessment   Education   IV's/Lines   Care plan review   I&O's   Chart check
Reassessment   Treatments   Skin   Nursing goals   General care   Sign off

Room:	Name:		Age/Sex:	Admit:

Code:	Allergies:	Isolation:

Attending:	Consults:

Diagnosis:	PMH:

Na:	RBC:	Meds:
K:	WBC:	
Ca:	Hgb:	
Mg:	Hct:	
Ph:	Platelets:	
Cl:	INR:	
Glu:	PTT:	
CO2:	BUN:	
	Creat:	

Diagnostics:	IV:	Fluids:

Vitals:		Intake	Output
T:			
P:			
R:			
BP:			
O2:			

Neuro:	Neuro/CIWA	Cardio/Tele:	Pain Assess:	Pain Reassess:	Blood Sugar:
Resp:	Lungs/O2	DVT Prophylaxis:			
GI: Diet: Last BM: GU:		Skin:	Edema: Mobility:	Notes:	

Assessment	Education	IV's/Lines	Care plan review	I&O's	Chart check
Reassessment	Treatments	Skin	Nursing goals	General care	Sign off

Room:	Name:		Age/Sex:	Admit:
Code:	Allergies:			Isolation:

Attending:	Consults:

Diagnosis:	PMH:

Na:	RBC:	Meds:
K:	WBC:	
Ca:	Hgb:	
Mg:	Hct:	
Ph:	Platelets:	
Cl:	INR:	
Glu:	PTT:	
CO2:	BUN:	
	Creat:	

Diagnostics:	IV:	Fluids:

Vitals:		Intake	Output
T:			
P:			
R:			
BP:			
O2:			

Neuro: Neuro/CIWA	Cardio/Tele:	Pain Assess:	Pain Reassess:	Blood Sugar:
Resp: Lungs/O2	DVT Prophylaxis:			
GI: Diet: Last BM:	Skin:	Edema:	Notes:	
GU:		Mobility:		

Assessment	Education	IV's/Lines	Care plan review	I&O's	Chart check
Reassessment	Treatments	Skin	Nursing goals	General care	Sign off

Room:	Name:		Age/Sex:	Admit:
Code:	Allergies:			Isolation:

Attending:	Consults:
Diagnosis:	PMH:

Na:	RBC:	Meds:
K:	WBC:	
Ca:	Hgb:	
Mg:	Hct:	
Ph:	Platelets:	
Cl:	INR:	
Glu:	PTT:	
CO2:	BUN:	
	Creat:	

Diagnostics:	IV:	Fluids:

Vitals:			Intake	Output
T:				
P:				
R:				
BP:				
O2:				

Neuro:	Neuro/CIWA	Cardio/Tele:	Pain Assess:	Pain Reassess:	Blood Sugar:
Resp:	Lungs/O2	DVT Prophylaxis:			
GI: Diet: Last BM:		Skin:	Edema:	Notes:	
GU:			Mobility:		

Assessment   Education   IV's/Lines   Care plan review   I&O's   Chart check
Reassessment   Treatments   Skin   Nursing goals   General care   Sign off

Room:	Name:		Age/Sex:	Admit:

Code:	Allergies:	Isolation:

Attending:	Consults:

Diagnosis:	PMH:

Na:	RBC:	Meds:
K:	WBC:	
Ca:	Hgb:	
Mg:	Hct:	
Ph:	Platelets:	
Cl:	INR:	
Glu:	PTT:	
CO2:	BUN:	
	Creat:	

Diagnostics:	IV:	Fluids:

Vitals:			Intake	Output
T:				
P:				
R:				
BP:				
O2:				

Neuro: Neuro/CIWA	Cardio/Tele:	Pain Assess:	Pain Reassess:	Blood Sugar:
Resp: Lungs/O2				
	DVT Prophylaxis:			
GI: Diet: Last BM:	Skin:	Edema:	Notes:	
GU:		Mobility:		

Assessment	Education	IV's/Lines	Care plan review	I&O's	Chart check
Reassessment	Treatments	Skin	Nursing goals	General care	Sign off

Room:	Name:			Age/Sex:	Admit:
Code:	Allergies:				Isolation:

Attending:	Consults:
Diagnosis:	PMH:

Na:	RBC:	Meds:
K:	WBC:	
Ca:	Hgb:	
Mg:	Hct:	
Ph:	Platelets:	
Cl:	INR:	
Glu:	PTT:	
CO2:	BUN:	
	Creat:	

Diagnostics:	IV:	Fluids:

Vitals:			Intake	Output
T:				
P:				
R:				
BP:				
O2:				

Neuro:	Neuro/CIWA	Cardio/Tele:	Pain Assess:	Pain Reassess:	Blood Sugar:
Resp:	Lungs/O2				
		DVT Prophylaxis:			
GI:		Skin:	Edema:	Notes:	
Diet:					
Last BM:			Mobility:		
GU:					

Assessment	Education	IV's/Lines	Care plan review	I&O's	Chart check
Reassessment	Treatments	Skin	Nursing goals	General care	Sign off

Room:	Name:		Age/Sex:	Admit:
Code:	Allergies:		Isolation:	

Attending:	Consults:

Diagnosis:	PMH:

Na:	RBC:	Meds:
K:	WBC:	
Ca:	Hgb:	
Mg:	Hct:	
Ph:	Platelets:	
Cl:	INR:	
Glu:	PTT:	
CO2:	BUN:	
	Creat:	

Diagnostics:	IV:	Fluids:

Vitals:			Intake	Output
T:				
P:				
R:				
BP:				
O2:				

Neuro:	Neuro/CIWA	Cardio/Tele:	Pain Assess:	Pain Reassess:	Blood Sugar:
Resp:	Lungs/O2	DVT Prophylaxis:			
GI: Diet: Last BM:		Skin:	Edema:	Notes:	
GU:			Mobility:		

Assessment	Education	IV's/Lines	Care plan review	I&O's	Chart check
Reassessment	Treatments	Skin	Nursing goals	General care	Sign off

Room:	Name:		Age/Sex:	Admit:
Code:	Allergies:			Isolation:

Attending:	Consults:

Diagnosis:	PMH:

Na:	RBC:	Meds:
K:	WBC:	
Ca:	Hgb:	
Mg:	Hct:	
Ph:	Platelets:	
Cl:	INR:	
Glu:	PTT:	
CO2:	BUN:	
	Creat:	

Diagnostics:	IV:	Fluids:

Vitals:			Intake	Output
T:				
P:				
R:				
BP:				
O2:				

Neuro:	Neuro/CIWA	Cardio/Tele:	Pain Assess:	Pain Reassess:	Blood Sugar:
Resp:	Lungs/O2	DVT Prophylaxis:			
GI: Diet: Last BM:		Skin:	Edema:	Notes:	
GU:			Mobility:		

Assessment	Education	IV's/Lines	Care plan review	I&O's	Chart check
Reassessment	Treatments	Skin	Nursing goals	General care	Sign off

Room:	Name:		Age/Sex:	Admit:

Code:	Allergies:		Isolation:

Attending:	Consults:

Diagnosis:	PMH:

Na:	RBC:	Meds:
K:	WBC:	
Ca:	Hgb:	
Mg:	Hct:	
Ph:	Platelets:	
Cl:	INR:	
Glu:	PTT:	
CO2:	BUN:	
	Creat:	

Diagnostics:	IV:	Fluids:

Vitals:			Intake	Output
T:				
P:				
R:				
BP:				
O2:				

Neuro:	Neuro/CIWA	Cardio/Tele:	Pain Assess:	Pain Reassess:	Blood Sugar:
Resp:	Lungs/O2				
		DVT Prophylaxis:			
GI:					
Diet:					
Last BM:		Skin:	Edema:	Notes:	
GU:			Mobility:		

Assessment	Education	IV's/Lines	Care plan review	I&O's	Chart check
Reassessment	Treatments	Skin	Nursing goals	General care	Sign off

Room:	Name:		Age/Sex:	Admit:
Code:	Allergies:			Isolation:

Attending:	Consults:
Diagnosis:	PMH:

Na:	RBC:	Meds:
K:	WBC:	
Ca:	Hgb:	
Mg:	Hct:	
Ph:	Platelets:	
Cl:	INR:	
Glu:	PTT:	
CO2:	BUN:	
	Creat:	

Diagnostics:	IV:	Fluids:

Vitals:			Intake	Output
T:				
P:				
R:				
BP:				
O2:				

Neuro:	Neuro/CIWA	Cardio/Tele:	Pain Assess:	Pain Reassess:	Blood Sugar:
Resp:	Lungs/O2	DVT Prophylaxis:			

GI:
  Diet:
  Last BM:
 	
GU:
		Skin:	Edema:
			
			Mobility:
				Notes:	

Assessment	Education	IV's/Lines	Care plan review	I&O's	Chart check
Reassessment	Treatments	Skin	Nursing goals	General care	Sign off

Room:	Name:		Age/Sex:	Admit:
Code:	Allergies:		Isolation:	

Attending:		Consults:

Diagnosis:		PMH:

Na:	RBC:	Meds:
K:	WBC:	
Ca:	Hgb:	
Mg:	Hct:	
Ph:	Platelets:	
Cl:	INR:	
Glu:	PTT:	
CO2:	BUN:	
	Creat:	

Diagnostics:		IV:	Fluids:

Vitals:			Intake	Output
T:				
P:				
R:				
BP:				
O2:				

Neuro:	Neuro/CIWA	Cardio/Tele:	Pain Assess:	Pain Reassess:	Blood Sugar:
Resp:	Lungs/O2	DVT Prophylaxis:			
GI: Diet: Last BM:					
GU:		Skin:	Edema: Mobility:	Notes:	

Assessment	Education	IV's/Lines	Care plan review	I&O's	Chart check
Reassessment	Treatments	Skin	Nursing goals	General care	Sign off

Room:	Name:			Age/Sex:	Admit:

Code:	Allergies:	Isolation:

Attending:	Consults:

Diagnosis:	PMH:

Na:	RBC:	Meds:
K:	WBC:	
Ca:	Hgb:	
Mg:	Hct:	
Ph:	Platelets:	
Cl:	INR:	
Glu:	PTT:	
CO2:	BUN:	
	Creat:	

Diagnostics:	IV:	Fluids:

Vitals:			Intake	Output
T:				
P:				
R:				
BP:				
O2:				

Neuro:	Neuro/CIWA	Cardio/Tele:	Pain Assess:	Pain Reassess:	Blood Sugar:
Resp:	Lungs/O2				
		DVT Prophylaxis:			
GI: Diet: Last BM:					
		Skin:	Edema:	Notes:	
GU:			Mobility:		

Assessment	Education	IV's/Lines	Care plan review	I&O's	Chart check
Reassessment	Treatments	Skin	Nursing goals	General care	Sign off

Room:	Name:		Age/Sex:	Admit:

Code:	Allergies:		Isolation:

Attending:	Consults:

Diagnosis:	PMH:

Na:	RBC:	Meds:
K:	WBC:	
Ca:	Hgb:	
Mg:	Hct:	
Ph:	Platelets:	
Cl:	INR:	
Glu:	PTT:	
CO2:	BUN:	
	Creat:	

Diagnostics:	IV:	Fluids:

Vitals:			Intake	Output
T:				
P:				
R:				
BP:				
O2:				

Neuro:	Neuro/CIWA	Cardio/Tele:	Pain Assess:	Pain Reassess:	Blood Sugar:
Resp:	Lungs/O2				
GI:		DVT Prophylaxis:			
Diet:					
Last BM:		Skin:	Edema:	Notes:	
GU:			Mobility:		

Assessment	Education	IV's/Lines	Care plan review	I&O's	Chart check
Reassessment	Treatments	Skin	Nursing goals	General care	Sign off

Room:	Name:		Age/Sex:	Admit:

Code:	Allergies:		Isolation:

Attending:	Consults:

Diagnosis:	PMH:

Na:	RBC:	Meds:
K:	WBC:	
Ca:	Hgb:	
Mg:	Hct:	
Ph:	Platelets:	
Cl:	INR:	
Glu:	PTT:	
CO2:	BUN:	
	Creat:	

Diagnostics:	IV:	Fluids:

Vitals:			Intake	Output
T:				
P:				
R:				
BP:				
O2:				

Neuro:	Neuro/CIWA	Cardio/Tele:	Pain Assess:	Pain Reassess:	Blood Sugar:
Resp:	Lungs/O2	DVT Prophylaxis:			
GI: Diet: Last BM:		Skin:	Edema:	Notes:	
GU:			Mobility:		

Assessment	Education	IV's/Lines	Care plan review	I&O's	Chart check
Reassessment	Treatments	Skin	Nursing goals	General care	Sign off

Room:	Name:		Age/Sex:	Admit:
Code:	Allergies:		Isolation:	

Attending:	Consults:
Diagnosis:	PMH:

Na:	RBC:	Meds:
K:	WBC:	
Ca:	Hgb:	
Mg:	Hct:	
Ph:	Platelets:	
Cl:	INR:	
Glu:	PTT:	
CO2:	BUN:	
	Creat:	

Diagnostics:	IV:	Fluids:

Vitals:			Intake	Output
T:				
P:				
R:				
BP:				
O2:				

Neuro:	Neuro/CIWA	Cardio/Tele:	Pain Assess:	Pain Reassess:	Blood Sugar:
Resp:	Lungs/O2	DVT Prophylaxis:			
GI: Diet: Last BM:		Skin:	Edema:	Notes:	
GU:			Mobility:		

Assessment	Education	IV's/Lines	Care plan review	I&O's	Chart check
Reassessment	Treatments	Skin	Nursing goals	General care	Sign off

Room:	Name:		Age/Sex:	Admit:

Code:	Allergies:	Isolation:

Attending:	Consults:

Diagnosis:	PMH:

Na:	RBC:	Meds:
K:	WBC:	
Ca:	Hgb:	
Mg:	Hct:	
Ph:	Platelets:	
Cl:	INR:	
Glu:	PTT:	
CO2:	BUN:	
	Creat:	

Diagnostics:	IV:	Fluids:

Vitals:			Intake	Output
T:				
P:				
R:				
BP:				
O2:				

Neuro:	Neuro/CIWA	Cardio/Tele:	Pain Assess:	Pain Reassess:	Blood Sugar:
Resp:	Lungs/O2	DVT Prophylaxis:			
GI: Diet: Last BM:		Skin:	Edema:	Notes:	
GU:			Mobility:		

Assessment	Education	IV's/Lines	Care plan review	I&O's	Chart check
Reassessment	Treatments	Skin	Nursing goals	General care	Sign off

Room:	Name:		Age/Sex:	Admit:
Code:	Allergies:			Isolation:

Attending:	Consults:
Diagnosis:	PMH:

Na:	RBC:	Meds:
K:	WBC:	
Ca:	Hgb:	
Mg:	Hct	
Ph:	Platelets:	
Cl:	INR:	
Glu:	PTT:	
CO2:	BUN:	
	Creat:	

Diagnostics:	IV:	Fluids:

Vitals:			Intake	Output
T:				
P:				
R:				
BP:				
O2:				

Neuro:	Neuro/CIWA	Cardio/Tele:	Pain Assess:	Pain Reassess:	Blood Sugar:
Resp:	Lungs/O2	DVT Prophylaxis:			
GI: Diet: Last BM:		Skin:	Edema:	Notes:	
GU:			Mobility:		

Assessment	Education	IV's/Lines	Care plan review	I&O's	Chart check
Reassessment	Treatments	Skin	Nursing goals	General care	Sign off

Room:	Name:			Age/Sex:	Admit:

Code:	Allergies:			Isolation:

Attending:

Consults:

Diagnosis:

PMH:

Na:	RBC:	Meds:
K:	WBC:	
Ca:	Hgb:	
Mg:	Hct:	
Ph:	Platelets:	
Cl:	INR:	
Glu:	PTT:	
CO2:	BUN:	
	Creat:	

Diagnostics:	IV:	Fluids:

Vitals:			Intake	Output
T:				
P:				
R:				
BP:				
O2:				

Neuro:	Neuro/CIWA	Cardio/Tele:	Pain Assess:	Pain Reassess:	Blood Sugar:
Resp:	Lungs/O2				
		DVT Prophylaxis:			
GI:					
Diet:					
Last BM:		Skin:	Edema:	Notes:	
GU:			Mobility:		

Assessment	Education	IV's/Lines	Care plan review	I&O's	Chart check
Reassessment	Treatments	Skin	Nursing goals	General care	Sign off

Room:	Name:		Age/Sex:	Admit:
Code:	Allergies:		Isolation:	
Attending:		Consults:		
Diagnosis:		PMH:		

Na:	RBC:	Meds:
K:	WBC:	
Ca:	Hgb:	
Mg:	Hct:	
Ph:	Platelets:	
Cl:	INR:	
Glu:	PTT:	
CO2:	BUN:	
	Creat:	

Diagnostics:	IV:	Fluids:

Vitals:			Intake	Output
T:				
P:				
R:				
BP:				
O2:				

Neuro:	Neuro/CIWA	Cardio/Tele:	Pain Assess:	Pain Reassess:	Blood Sugar:
Resp:	Lungs/O2	DVT Prophylaxis:			

GI:
  Diet:
  Last BM:
 	
GU:
		Skin:	Edema:
			
			Mobility:
				Notes:	

Assessment   Education   IV's/Lines   Care plan review   I&O's   Chart check
Reassessment   Treatments   Skin   Nursing goals   General care   Sign off

Room:	Name:		Age/Sex:	Admit:
Code:	Allergies:		Isolation:	

Attending:	Consults:
Diagnosis:	PMH:

Na:	RBC:	Meds:
K:	WBC:	
Ca:	Hgb:	
Mg:	Hct:	
Ph:	Platelets:	
Cl:	INR:	
Glu:	PTT:	
CO2:	BUN:	
	Creat:	

Diagnostics:	IV:	Fluids:

Vitals:			Intake	Output
T:				
P:				
R:				
BP:				
O2:				

Neuro:	Neuro/CIWA	Cardio/Tele:	Pain Assess:	Pain Reassess:	Blood Sugar:
Resp:	Lungs/O2	DVT Prophylaxis:			
GI: Diet: Last BM: GU:		Skin:	Edema: Mobility:	Notes:	

Assessment	Education	IV's/Lines	Care plan review	I&O's	Chart check
Reassessment	Treatments	Skin	Nursing goals	General care	Sign off

Room:	Name:		Age/Sex:	Admit:
Code:	Allergies:			Isolation:

Attending:	Consults:
Diagnosis:	PMH:

Na:	RBC:	Meds:
K:	WBC:	
Ca:	Hgb:	
Mg:	Hct:	
Ph:	Platelets:	
Cl:	INR:	
Glu:	PTT:	
CO2:	BUN:	
	Creat:	

Diagnostics:	IV:	Fluids:

Vitals:			Intake	Output
T:				
P:				
R:				
BP:				
O2:				

Neuro:	Neuro/CIWA	Cardio/Tele:	Pain Assess:	Pain Reassess:	Blood Sugar:
Resp:	Lungs/O2				
		DVT Prophylaxis:			
GI: Diet: Last BM:					
		Skin:	Edema:	Notes:	
GU:			Mobility:		

Assessment	Education	IV's/Lines	Care plan review	I&O's	Chart check
Reassessment	Treatments	Skin	Nursing goals	General care	Sign off

Room:	Name:		Age/Sex:	Admit:

Code:	Allergies:	Isolation:

Attending:	Consults:

Diagnosis:	PMH:

Na:	RBC:	Meds:
K:	WBC:	
Ca:	Hgb:	
Mg:	Hct:	
Ph:	Platelets:	
Cl:	INR:	
Glu:	PTT:	
CO2:	BUN:	
	Creat:	

Diagnostics:	IV:	Fluids:

Vitals:			Intake	Output
T:				
P:				
R:				
BP:				
O2:				

Neuro:	Neuro/CIWA	Cardio/Tele:	Pain Assess:	Pain Reassess:	Blood Sugar:
Resp:	Lungs/O2	DVT Prophylaxis:			
GI: Diet: Last BM: GU:		Skin:	Edema: Mobility:	Notes:	

Assessment   Education   IV's/Lines   Care plan review   I&O's   Chart check

Reassessment   Treatments   Skin   Nursing goals   General care   Sign off

Made in the USA
Monee, IL
10 September 2022